Milady Standard Esthetics: Advanced Exam Review

Second Edition

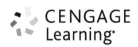

Australia • Brazil • Japan • Korea • Mexico • Singapore • Spain • United Kingdom • United States

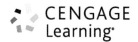
CENGAGE
Learning·

Milady Standard Esthetics: Advanced Exam Review, Second Edition
Milady

President, Milady:
Dawn Gerrain

Director of Content and Business Development:
Sandra Bruce

Associate Acquisitions Editor:
Philip Mandl

Product Manager:
Maria Moffre-Barnes

Editorial Assistant:
Elizabeth A. Edwards

Director of Marketing and Training:
Gerard McAvey

Senior Production Director:
Wendy A. Troeger

Production Manager:
Sherondra Thedford

Senior Content Project Manager:
Angela Sheehan

Senior Art Director:
Benjamin Gleeksman

© 2013 Milady, a part of Cengage Learning.

ALL RIGHTS RESERVED. No part of this work covered by the copyright herein may be reproduced, transmitted, stored, or used in any form or by any means graphic, electronic, or mechanical, including but not limited to photocopying, recording, scanning, digitizing, taping, Web distribution, information networks, or information storage and retrieval systems, except as permitted under Section 107 or 108 of the 1976 United States Copyright Act, without the prior written permission of the publisher.

For product information and technology assistance, contact us at **Professional & Career Group Customer Support, 1-800-648-7450**

For permission to use material from this text or product, submit all requests online at **cengage.com/permissions.** Further permissions questions can be e-mailed to **permissionrequest@cengage.com.**

Library of Congress Control Number: 2011943910

ISBN-13: 978-1-111-13912-4

ISBN-10: 1-111-13912-1

Milady
5 Maxwell Drive
Clifton Park, NY 12065-2919
USA

Cengage Learning products are represented in Canada by Nelson Education, Ltd.

For your lifelong learning solutions, visit **milady.cengage.com**

Visit our corporate website at **cengage.com.**

Notice to the Reader
Publisher does not warrant or guarantee any of the products described herein or perform any independent analysis in connection with any of the product information contained herein. Publisher does not assume, and expressly disclaims, any obligation to obtain and include information other than that provided to it by the manufacturer. The reader is expressly warned to consider and adopt all safety precautions that might be indicated by the activities described herein and to avoid all potential hazards. By following the instructions contained herein, the reader willingly assumes all risks in connection with such instructions. The publisher makes no representations or warranties of any kind, including but not limited to, the warranties of fitness for particular purpose or merchantability, nor are any such representations implied with respect to the material set forth herein, and the publisher takes no responsibility with respect to such material. The publisher shall not be liable for any special, consequential, or exemplary damages resulting, in whole or part, from the readers' use of, or reliance upon, this material.

Printed at CLDPC, USA, 09-18

Milady Standard Esthetics: Advanced Exam Review

Foreword

Milady Standard Esthetics: Advanced Exam Review follows the type of skin care questions most frequently used by states and by the national testing, conducted under the auspices of the National-Interstate Council of State Boards of Cosmetology.

This review book is designed to be of major assistance to students in preparing for the state license examinations and future career path. The exclusive concentration on multiple-choice test items reflects the fact that all state board examinations and national testing examinations are confined to this type of question.

Questions on the state board examinations in different states will not be exactly like these and may not touch upon all the information covered in this review. But students who diligently study and practice their work as taught in the classroom and who use this book for test preparation and review should receive higher grades on both classroom and license examinations.

The answers to the questions are found at the end of the book.

Part 1: Orientation

CHAPTER 1—CHANGES IN ESTHETICS

1. What generation's desire, willingness, and financial ability to lengthen youthfulness have had a huge effect on the industry?
   a. baby boomers
   b. the World War II generation
   c. Generation X
   d. Generation Y _____

2. What can estheticians do if they constantly seek out education, encourage research, and take the time to root out the facts?
   a. guarantee financial stability
   b. successfully meet challenges
   c. guarantee perfect results for clients
   d. become beauty-industry celebrities _____

3. What is true of most of the spa treatments provided today?
   a. they are derivations of treatments introduced in the 20th century
   b. they are completely new concepts unrelated to previous treatments
   c. they are derivations of ancient treatments
   d. they are exactly the same as treatments provided in ancient times _____

4. What is **NOT** one of the types of bathhouses found in ancient Rome?
   a. balnea
   b. balnea private
   c. balnea public
   d. balnea professional _____

5. What change in bathing habits occurred as a result of the fall of the Roman empire?
   a. public bathing was prohibited by the religious culture
   b. Roman bathing habits were continued in all countries
   c. bathhouses were turned into exercise retreats, the precursors of gyms
   d. daily bathing in the home became commonplace _____

6. What term refers to medicinal process of bloodletting, which was performed at baths during medieval times?
   a. lobotomy
   b. phlebotomy
   c. rhytidectomy
   d. rhinoplasty _____

7. What trend resulted from the common public fear during the
   Renaissance that the bathhouse was the cause of diseases such as
   syphilis and leprosy?
   a. the use of scalding-hot water in baths
   b. the use of bleach in bathwater
   c. a preference for showering over bathing
   d. a decline in the use of public baths ____

8. When did the philosophy of drinking mineral water, in addition to
   bathing in it, become commonplace?
   a. Renaissance   c. Elizabethan era
   b. Victorian era   d. medieval times ____

9. What did the French use cold springs for during the seventeenth
   century?
   a. bathing   c. water-based massage
   b. drinking therapies   d. mud baths ____

10. What did the 19th-century Bavarian monk Father Sebastian Kneipp
    believe that using water to eliminate waste from the body would do?
    a. encourage relaxation   c. improve social stature
    b. provide spiritual balance d. cure disease ____

11. What types of businesses were introduced the United States between
    the mid-1800s and the beginning of the depression in the 1930s?
    a. day spas   c. wellness centers
    b. spa resorts   d. massage parlors ____

12. What is **NOT** one of the new treatments that became popular in the
    United States after World War II?
    a. health and exercise regimens c. mud therapy
    b. bloodletting   d. hydrotherapy ____

13. What is the fastest-growing global market for spas?
    a. South America   c. Europe
    b. North America   d. Asia ____

14. What is true about the amount of training and education estheticians
    need?
    a. everyone agrees on the same rules
    b. each professional in the esthetics field requires a postgraduate
       degree
    c. no special training is required for working in the esthetics field
    d. this has long been up for debate ____

15. What caused the demand for solid, advanced esthetics education to skyrocket?
    a. the medical profession's embrace of esthetics
    b. sales generated by celebrity endorsements of beauty products
    c. government regulations that cracked down on untrained estheticians
    d. marketing opportunities created by the spread of the Internet ____

16. Why would a doctor hire the better-trained of two candidates for an esthetics position?
    a. the better-trained candidate is eager to pay off student loans
    b. less time is involved training the better-trained candidate
    c. the better-trained candidate can prescribe medications
    d. the better-trained candidate can perform surgical procedures ____

17. What is **NOT** one of the primary functions of an esthetician?
    a. performing facials
    b. performing skin treatments
    c. diagnosing medical conditions
    d. applying cosmetics ____

18. What is **NOT** one of the skill sets required for estheticians?
    a. ability to control inventory
    b. ability to perform chemistry
    c. ability to plan marketing
    d. ability to build a client base ____

19. What profession requires the skill sets of loving fashion and being able to guide clients into adapting trends for individual use?
    a. medical esthetician   c. salon manager
    b. esthetics instructor   d. makeup artist ____

20. What is one of the most common services offered by permanent makeup artists?
    a. eyeliner   c. lipstick
    b. blush   d. concealer ____

21. What profession requires knowledge of the technical skills needed to implant color into the skin so that it will stay?
    a. bridal makeup artist   c. theatrical makeup artist
    b. permanent makeup artist   d. advertising makeup artist ____

22. What should an esthetician seeking work in the medical field have a solid knowledge of, in addition to his or her knowledge of advanced skin care?
    a. color theory
    b. fashion trends
    c. medical terminology
    d. medical billing ____

23. What type of makeup techniques should estheticians in the medical field understand?
    a. corrective
    b. theatrical
    c. bridal
    d. advertising ____

24. What do estheticians and makeup artists for resorts and cruise lines offer in addition to personal services?
    a. demonstrations
    b. professional training
    c. medical services
    d. full-body massage ____

25. What is **NOT** one of the skills required for success as a salon or spa owner?
    a. strong writing abilities
    b. financial management
    c. marketing
    d. people management ____

26. What is the **MAIN** reason most esthetics instructors attend workshops and conferences?
    a. to get free product samples
    b. to make new personal friends
    c. to keep their knowledge up to date
    d. to look for new jobs ____

27. What is a special requirement of those working as manufacturer/sales representatives?
    a. impeccable appearance
    b. advanced college degree
    c. extensive scientific knowledge
    d. ability to speak several languages ____

28. What do many cosmetics lines do for licensed estheticians because they have realized how much professional training benefit the lines' clients?
    a. pay for the estheticians' training
    b. pay higher wages than salons
    c. build their own training centers
    d. lobby for relaxed licensing rules ____

29. What is **NOT** one of the responsibilities of an assistant buyer?
    a. placing orders   c. tracking inventory
    b. estimating product needs   d. helping the buyer   _____

30. What must a manager be able to do?
    a. motivate the sales staff
    b. guarantee continued employment
    c. help staff with personal problems
    d. apply permanent makeup   _____

31. What professional field should someone seeking work as a beauty
    editor or columnist have experience in?
    a. education   c. journalism
    b. medicine   d. sales   _____

32. What is a special skill required for work as a state licensing inspector
    or examiner?
    a. color theory   c. fashion knowledge
    b. diplomacy   d. salesmanship   _____

33. What step of critical thinking involves evaluating how a problem may
    have been caused?
    a. clarifying the concern
    b. gathering the facts
    c. examining the evidence
    d. defining solutions and outcomes   _____

34. What step of critical thinking involves considering different points of
    view?
    a. defining solutions and outcomes   c. examining the evidence
    b. gathering the facts   d. clarifying the concern   _____

35. What does the "S" stand for in the term "SOAP notes," which refers
    to a method of documenting the critical-thinking process?
    a. salon   c. subjective
    b. selective   d. spa   _____

Part 2: General Sciences

CHAPTER 2—INFECTION CONTROL

1. What is a disease resulting from human immunodeficiency virus?
   a. cancer
   b. leukemia
   c. AIDS
   d. tuberculosis

   _C_

2. What term refers to the rapid-onset, short-term initial stage of disease?
   a. pathogen
   b. acute
   c. chronic
   d. sharp

   _B_

3. What does the term "antibacterial" mean?
   a. infected with bacteria
   b. destroying or stopping the growth of bacteria
   c. capable of carrying bacteria
   d. indication that bacteria is multiplying on a surface

   _B_

4. What fluid is **NOT** considered contaminated and/or infectious under standard precautions?
   a. blood
   b. saliva
   c. sweat
   d. pus

   _C_

5. What term refers to any object that can penetrate the skin?
   a. hazard
   b. acute
   c. chronic
   d. sharp

   _D_

6. What is the correct term for a plan for avoiding potential exposure and for dealing with it should exposure occur?
   a. exposure plan
   b. hazard plan
   c. safety plan
   d. pathogen plan

   _C_

7. What term indicates that something is transmitted through direct blood-to-blood contact?
   a. bloodborne
   b. contagious
   c. opportunistic
   d. pathogenic

   _A_

8. What is mechanical irritation?
   a. the process of becoming immune to a pathogen
   b. tissue damage due to repeated physical contact to the tissue
   c. a microscopic organism capable of producing disease
   d. the rapid-onset, short-term initial stage of disease

   _B_

9. How are transient microorganisms removed from the hands?
   a. exposure to sunlight
   b. exposure to radiation
   c. hand washing
   d. chemical sterilization of the hands

   c

10. What are microorganisms that are often present on the surface of the human body?
    a. transient microorganisms   c. bacterial spores
    b. opportunistic bacteria   d. resident microorganisms

    D

11. What is a pathogen?
    a. a reproductive cell produced by plants and some protozoa
    b. a microorganism or substance capable of producing disease
    c. a membrane that lines a passage or cavity that communicates with air
    d. an infection acquired in a hospital or other health care environment

    B

12. What term describes the risks involved in piercing mucous membranes or the skin through needlesticks, bites, cuts, and abrasions?
    a. parenteral hazards   c. mechanical irritation
    b. endogenous infections   d. occupational exposure

    A

13. What term refers to any living thing, plant or animal?
    a. organism   c. pathogen
    b. microorganism   d. bacteria

    A

14. What are bacteria that will not cause harm when on a healthy host, but can cause infection and disease once they have entered the skin?
    a. occupational bacteria   c. resident bacteria
    b. transient bacteria   d. opportunistic bacteria

    D

15. Where would one acquire a nosocomial infection?
    a. hospital   c. shopping mall
    b. school   d. park

    A

16. What is **NOT** one of the components of a mucous membrane?
    a. epithelium   c. connective tissue
    b. basement membrane   d. attic membrane

    D

17. What is the correct term for the process of becoming immune or rendering a person immune to a pathogen?
    a. regeneration
    c. sterilization
    b. immunization
    d. disinfection

    B

18. What term refers to devices that isolate or remove bloodborne pathogen hazards from the workplace?
    a. engineering controls
    c. cleansers
    b. standard precautions
    d. disinfectants

    A

19. What is an infection that occurs when bacteria travel from a site where they were harmless to a site where they cause infection?
    a. mechanical infection
    c. resident infection
    b. nosocomial infection
    d. endogenous infection

    D

20. What is **NOT** one of the definitions of the word "contaminate"?
    a. to render impure
    c. to isolate or remove
    b. to soil, stain, or pollute
    d. to render unfit for use

    C

21. What does the term "asepsis" mean?
    a. destroying or stopping the growth of bacteria
    b. a condition free from germs and any form of life
    c. transmitted through direct blood-to-blood contact
    d. rendering a person immune to a pathogen

    B

22. What variety of hepatitis is transmitted by drinking water or eating food contaminated with fecal matter containing the virus?
    a. hepatitis A
    c. hepatitis C
    b. hepatitis B
    d. hepatitis D

    A

23. What variety of hepatitis can be treated without the use of interferon?
    a. hepatitis A
    c. hepatitis C
    b. hepatitis B
    d. hepatitis D

    A

24. What is **NOT** one of the times when hand washing should be performed?
    a. when hands are visibly soiled
    c. upon arriving at work
    b. after gloving
    d. before eating or drinking

    B

25. What federal agency would send inspectors to a salon because an accident has occurred in which three or more employees were injured?
    a. Centers for Disease Control and Prevention (CDC)
    b. United States Department of Agriculture (USDA)
    c. Occupational Safety and Health Administration (OSHA)
    d. Food and Drug Administration (FDA)   *C*

26. What should you do if you are visited by an inspector from OSHA?
    a. panic
    b. volunteer unsolicited information
    c. answer questions deceptively
    d. write down the inspector's name   *D*

27. What is the second link in the chain of infection?
    a. infectious agent
    b. reservoir where the agent resides
    c. portal of entry
    d. susceptible host to infect   *B*

28. What is the second-to-last link in the chain of infection?
    a. susceptible host to infect   c. portal of entry
    b. reservoir where the agent resides d. infectious agent *C*

29. Why should you follow OSHA guidelines if you are a sole proprietor and work alone?
    a. you are legally required to do so
    b. to increase financial profitability
    c. so you can include the OSHA logo in your advertisements
    d. to live a long and healthy life   *D*

30. What is **NOT** one of the means by which human immunodeficiency virus (HIV) is spread from an infected person to a noninfected person?
    a. contact with sweat   c. contact with saliva
    b. contact with blood   d. contact with broken skin *D*

31. What organ is most often affected by the highly infectious disease tuberculosis?
    a. heart   c. kidneys
    b. lungs   d. stomach   *A*

10

32. Why have many states passed laws that prohibit spitting on sidewalks?
    a. because spitting is the most common means of spreading HIV
    b. there are no such laws in the United States
    c. because vapors from saliva cause many skin diseases
    d. because tuberculosis can live on a sidewalk in sputum for six months

    D

33. What is **NOT** one of the forms in which methicillin-resistant Staphylococcus aureus (MRSA) skin infections can present themselves?
    a. cellulitis   c. vitiligo
    b. impetigo   d. carbuncles

    C

34. What is one of the steps you can take to minimize the spread of MRSA?
    a. drying hands with reusable towels
    b. only using gloves for extractions
    c. cleaning and reusing materials that come in contact with blood
    d. cleaning and disinfecting all work surfaces

    D

35. What mode of transmission involves contact with an animal, insect, or parasite that transports infection by biting the host or by depositing feces or eggs in broken skin?
    a. direct contact   c. airborne transmission
    b. vector transmission   d. indirect contact

    B

CHAPTER 3—ADVANCED HISTOLOGY OF THE CELL AND THE SKIN

1. What is a protein in a muscle fiber that, together with myocin, is responsible for contraction and relaxation?
   a. actin
   b. basophil
   c. corium
   d. dendrite

   A

2. What is the process that requires expenditure of adenosine triphosphate (ATP) energy to move molecules across a cell membrane?
   a. cell cycle
   b. active transport
   c. epidermal growth factor
   d. fibroblast growth factor

   B

3. What are junctions that provide strong mechanical attachments between adjacent cells?
   a. gap junctions
   b. tight junctions
   c. adherens junctions
   d. loose junctions

   C

4. What is a zygote?
   a. intermediate filament found in fibroblasts
   b. protein that forms parts of the microtubes
   c. protein that binds to cyclin and CdK
   d. diploid cell produced by the fusion of an egg and sperm

   D

5. What is vimentin?
   a. intermediate filament found in fibroblasts
   b. protein responsible for contraction and relaxation
   c. fluid-filled or yolk-filled cavity surrounded by a blastoderm
   d. proteoglycan found in the dermis

   A

6. What are membrane-bound compartments within some eukaryotic cells that can serve a variety of secretory, excretory, and storage functions?
   a. proteoglycans
   b. vacuoles
   c. plaques
   d. microfilaments

   B

7. What organic acids form the building blocks of proteins?
   a. free fatty acids
   b. amino acids
   c. hyaluronic acids
   d. hypochlorous acids

   B

8. What is the scientific name for chlorine bleach?
   a. hypochlorous acid
   b. free fatty acid
   c. amino acid
   d. hyaluronic acid

   A

9. What is the study of tiny structures found in living tissues?
   a. biology
   b. anatomy
   c. physiology
   d. histology

   D

10. What is a phospholipid bilayer in living organisms that is impregnated with protein and certain other compounds and that is differentially permeable?
    a. membrane
    b. muscle
    c. organ
    d. system

    A

11. What is apoptosis?
    a. fluid- or yolk-filled cavity
    b. genetically determined cell death
    c. lipid component of the stratum corneum
    d. proteoglycan found in the dermis

    B

12. What term refers to the system that controls involuntary functions of the circulatory, respiratory, endocrine, and digestive systems?
    a. involuntary nervous system
    b. automatic nervous system
    c. passive nervous system
    d. programmed nervous system

    B

13. What is a protein important in stabilizing cell adherence to avoid abnormal spread of cells?
    a. basophil
    b. keratin sulfate
    c. zygote
    d. catenin

    D

14. What is a region of actual fusion of cell membranes between two adjacent cells?
    a. adherens junction
    b. loose junction
    c. tight junction
    d. gap junction

    C

15. What is a superoxide?
    a. unstable, reactive single oxygen atom
    b. special protein on a cell's surface that binds to specific ligands
    c. elastin-type fiber found in the dermis
    d. enzyme used in the killing action of neutrophils

    A

16. What is a layer of the ectoderm germ layer that provides most of the central nervous system?
    a. nuclear membrane
    b. pluripotential stem cell
    c. polychromatic normoblast
    d. neural tube

    D

17. What term refers to a cell capable of multiple divisions?
    a. stem cell   c. mast cell
    b. senescent cell   d. Langerhans cell

    A

18. What cells are also known as "mother cells"?
    a. mast cells   c. Langerhans cells
    b. stem cells   d. senescent cells

    B

19. What are circular or ovoid structures with a distinct connective tissue capsule that can transmit touch, pressure, and cold?
    a. Langerhans cells   c. Meissner's corpuscles
    b. basophilic normoblasts d. senescent cells

    C

20. What is a process that uses oxygen in the killing action of neutrophils?
    a. respiratory burst
    b. cell cycle
    c. reflex arc
    d. maturation promotion factor

    A

21. What is an enzyme capable of dissolving and digesting many types of biochemicals?
    a. macrophage   c. integrin
    b. lysozyme   d. humoral

    B

22. What is cholesterol?
    a. lipid component of the stratum corneum
    b. complex carbohydrate in the dermis
    c. elastin-type fiber found in the dermis
    d. deep primary germ layer of the embryo

    A

23. What does the term "efferent" mean?
    a. supportive cells closely associated with neurons
    b. leading or conveying away from some organ
    c. pertaining to an endocrine solution
    d. composed of keratinocyte

    B

24. What type of collagen is found in skin, bone, and tendon?
    a. type I   c. type III
    b. type II   d. type IV

    A

25. Where in the body is type V collagen found?
    a. skin   c. tendon
    b. fribrillar cartilage   d. interstitial tissue

    D

26. How many types of collagen are there?
    a. five
    b. seven
    c. 11
    d. 15

    _C_

27. What are cells that serve as managers and direct the immune response?
    a. B cells
    b. helper T cells
    c. M cells
    d. dendritic cells

    _B_

28. What is a complex process that reproduces the critical information in each cell for proper functioning and reproduction?
    a. cell-mediated immunity
    b. epidermal growth factor
    c. DNA synthesis
    d. fibroblast growth factor

    _C_

29. What are nerve endings in the skin without myelin sheaths?
    a. nerve fibers
    b. nerve impulses
    c. mandibular nerves
    d. free nerve terminals

    _D_

30. What cranial nerve is the maxillary nerve a branch of?
    a. first
    b. second
    c. fourth
    d. fifth

    _D_

31. What are cells that are programmed to recognize and respond to a pathogen once it has invaded and been repelled?
    a. memory T cells
    b. helper T cells
    c. cytotoxic T cells
    d. recognition T cells

    _A_

32. What is the fatty material forming the medullary sheath of nerve fibers?
    a. mitosis
    b. monocyte
    c. myosin
    d. myelin

    _D_

33. What is the basic unit of the nervous system, consisting of a cell body, a nucleus, dendrites, and an axon?
    a. muscle
    b. fiber
    c. tissue
    d. neuron

    _D_

16

34. Where are organelles found?
    a. cytoplasm of eukaryotic cells
    b. cell membrane of eukaryotic cells
    c. cytoplasm of cytotoxic cells
    d. cell membrane of cytotoxic cells

    _A_

35. What is a protein that initiates part of the cellular division known as mitosis?
    a. epidermal growth factor
    b. fibroblast growth factor
    c. maturation promoting factor
    d. cellular division factor

    _C_

CHAPTER 4—HORMONES

1. What term refers to the daily biochemical patterns of the body?
   a. circadian rhythm
   b. endometrium
   c. hormone replacement therapy
   d. thyrotoxicosis _____

2. What are coiled structures attached to the hair follicles found in the underarm and genital areas?
   a. pituitary glands   c. pineal glands
   b. apocrine glands   d. thyroid glands _____

3. What is a temporary endocrine structure that develops from the ovarian follicle during the menstrual cycle?
   a. striae distensae   c. corpus luteum
   b. linea nigra   d. progesterone _____

4. What hormone regulates absorption of calcium and vitamin D?
   a. androgen   c. melatonin
   b. estrogen   d. calcitonin _____

5. What are corticoids?
   a. steroid hormones produced by the adrenal cortex
   b. coiled structures attached to hair follicles in the genital areas
   c. steroid hormones that help regulate blood sugar
   d. secretions produced by the endocrine glands _____

6. What is a major steroid hormone, often called the stress hormone, that is produced in the adrenal cortex?
   a. cortisol   c. androgen
   b. estrogen   d. calcitonin _____

7. What is a disease that results when the pancreas does not secrete enough insulin?
   a. sickle cell anemia   c. leukemia
   b. diabetes   d. pneumonia _____

8. What are ductless glands that release hormonal secretions directly into the bloodstream?
   a. pineal glands   c. thyroid glands
   b. thymus glands   d. endocrine glands _____

9. What is the body system of ductless glands that secrete or produce hormones?
   a. endocrine system
   b. lymphatic system
   c. integumentary system
   d. circulatory system
   _____

10. What is the endometrium?
    a. outer membrane of the uterus
    b. inner membrane of the uterus
    c. outer membrane of the cervix
    d. inner membrane of the cervix
    _____

11. What is a steroid made from the hormone estrogen that gives women female characteristics?
    a. estradiol
    b. estriol
    c. endometrium
    d. endocrine
    _____

12. What hormone gives women female characteristics?
    a. progestin
    b. mineralcorticoid
    c. glucocorticoid
    d. estrogen
    _____

13. What hormone secreted by the pituitary gland causes the development of the egg (also known as the ovum)?
    a. epidermal growth factor (EGF)
    b. follicle-stimulating hormone (FSH)
    c. insulin-like growth factor (IGF)
    d. prolactin releasing hormone (PRH)
    _____

14. What is an itching and tingling feeling of the skin experienced by some women during menopause?
    a. thyrotoxicosis
    b. formication
    c. myxedema
    d. endometrium
    _____

15. What are glucocorticodes?
    a. steroid hormones that help regulate sugar
    b. chemicals that cause the glands to make hormones
    c. ductless glands that release hormonal secretions
    d. steroid hormones that help regulate blood minerals
    _____

16. What is an autoimmune disease in which the immune system attacks the thyroid so that it cannot function properly?
    a. AIDS
    b. Hashimoto's thyroiditis
    c. diabetes
    d. chronic lymphocytic leukemia
    _____

17. What structures on the cell membrane receive and accept hormones and, in turn, produce other biochemicals that cause or stimulate different functions in the cells?
    a. trophic hormones
    b. neurohormones
    c. hormone receptors
    d. leutenizing hormones

    ____

18. What are secretions produced by one of the endocrine glands that are the internal messengers for most of the body's systems?
    a. white blood cells
    b. red blood cells
    c. enzymes
    d. hormones

    ____

19. What gland manufactures hormones that stimulate the pituitary gland to make other hormones?
    a. hypothalamus
    b. thyroid
    c. pancreas
    d. ovary

    ____

20. What term refers to redness and bumpiness common on the cheeks or upper arms that is caused by blocked hair follicles?
    a. pseudofolliculitis
    b. keratosis pilaris
    c. hyperpigmentation
    d. hypopigmentation

    ____

21. What is a hormone that causes ovulation (the release of the egg from the ovary) in females and causes the testes in males to manufacture testosterone?
    a. trophic hormone
    b. neurohormone
    c. leutenizing hormone
    d. hormone receptor

    ____

22. What is a specialized hormone secreted by the pineal gland that helps regulate the body's responses to different levels of light?
    a. calcitonin
    b. cortisol
    c. estrone
    d. melatonin

    ____

23. What term refers to the first menstrual period?
    a. menarche
    b. melasma
    c. menopause
    d. myxedema

    ____

24. What is the process by which the female body rids itself of an unused ovum and the accompanying endometrium?
    a. menopause
    b. menstruation
    c. melasma
    d. myxedema

    ____

25. What are mineralcorticoids?
    a. chemicals that cause glands to make hormones
    b. the organs of the male reproductive system
    c. steroid hormones that help regulate blood minerals
    d. ductless glands that release hormonal secretions ____

26. What is a hyperthyroid condition in which the skin on the shins becomes thick and red-brown with a bumpy texture?
    a. eczema   c. hyperpigmentation
    b. rosacea   d. myxedema   ____

27. What hormones are secreted by the hypothalamus and control many pituitary hormone secretions?
    a. neurohormones   c. hormone receptors
    b. trophic hormones   d. leutenizing hormones ____

28. What is a thinning of the bones that leaves the bones fragile and prone to fractures?
    a. diabetes   c. leukemia
    b. osteoporosis   d. anemia   ____

29. What is the function of the parathyroid gland?
    a. serving as the "brain" of the endocrine system
    b. regulating cellular and body metabolism
    c. regulating calcium and phosphates in the bloodstream
    d. unknown but thought to be related to the sex hormones ____

30. What is a hormonal disorder in women caused by excessive presence of androgens?
    a. premenstrual syndrome
    b. osteoporosis
    c. circadian rhythm
    d. polycystic ovarian syndrome ____

31. What is a hormone that helps prepare the uterus for pregnancy and is an important hormone in the menstrual cycle?
    a. progesterone   c. testosterone
    b. androgen   d. calcitonin   ____

32. What is a hormone manufactured by the ovaries that helps enlarge the pelvic opening during childbirth?
    a. calcitonin   c. androgen
    b. relaxin   d. progesterone   ____

33. What does the term "secreted" mean?
    a. issued from an infected follicle
    b. transported by the cardiovascular system
    c. synthesized or released by various cells or organs
    d. absorbed into the skin _____

34. What is the male hormone responsible for development of typical male characteristics?
    a. estrogen
    c. thyroxine
    b. progesterone
    d. testosterone _____

35. What term refers to the group of clinical symptoms associated with hyperthyroidism?
    a. thyrotoxicosis
    c. striae distensae
    b. trophic hormones
    d. neurohormones _____

CHAPTER 5—ANATOMY AND PHYSIOLOGY: MUSCLES AND NERVES

1. What neurotransmitter has the primary function of mediating synaptic activity of the nervous system and skeletal muscles?
    a. acetylcholine
    b. brachialis
    c. erector spinae
    d. frenulum
    _____

2. What term refers to smaller muscles that keep the legs together during most physical activity?
    a. arrector pili muscles
    b. adductor muscles
    c. external obliques
    d. internal obliques
    _____

3. What is an antagonist?
    a. something that transmits sound, heat, light, or energy
    b. something that changes shape and returns to its original form
    c. something that opposes the action of another
    d. something that excites or incites an organ to function
    _____

4. What does "anterior" mean?
    a. front
    b. back
    c. top
    d. bottom
    _____

5. What strong, thick, and flat connective tissue serves as fascia to bind muscles together or as tendon to attach muscle to bone?
    a. rectus abdominis
    b. latissimus dorsi
    c. gastrocnemius
    d. aponeurosis
    _____

6. What smooth muscles are attached to hair follicles and cause the hair to stand erect when they contract?
    a. adductor muscles
    b. arrector pili muscles
    c. internal obliques
    d. external obliques
    _____

7. Where in the body is the biceps brachii muscle found?
    a. chest
    b. thigh
    c. upper arm
    d. back of the neck
    _____

8. What term refers to the movement of a limb or extremity in which the distal end describes a circle while the proximal end remains fixed?
    a. abduction
    b. adduction
    c. eversion
    d. circumduction
    _____

9. What term means "away from, or farthest from, a point of origin or the midline or center"?
   a. distal
   b. ala
   c. nare
   d. fascia ____

10. What is the erector spinae?
   a. flaring cartilaginous expansion on each side of the nare
   b. set of three muscles that run along either side of the spinal column
   c. important muscle for the arm's ability to flex at the elbow
   d. any of three muscles of the posterior thigh ____

11. What term refers to any muscle that allows for extension of a body part, such the muscle that extends the index finger?
   a. distal
   b. fascia
   c. extensor
   d. posterior ____

12. What is a thin, long muscle that runs the length of the side of the tibialis anterior muscle?
   a. rectus abdominis
   b. latissimus dorsi
   c. gastrocnemius
   d. extensor digitorium longus ____

13. What muscles are responsible for the movement of the vertebrae and rotation of the torso?
   a. external obliques
   b. internal obliques
   c. adductor muscles
   d. arrector pili muscles ____

14. What is a movement allowed by certain joints that decreases the angle between two adjoining bones, such as bending the elbow?
   a. flexion
   b. abduction
   c. eversion
   d. rotation ____

15. What is a fold of mucous membrane that connects two parts, as between the lips and the gums, one being more or less movable?
   a. fascia
   b. frenulum
   c. ala
   d. nare ____

16. Where is the gastrocnemius muscle located?
   a. hip
   b. ankle
   c. calf
   d. thigh ____

17. What part of the body gets its exterior contours from the gluteal muscles?
    a. breasts
    b. face
    c. abdomen
    d. buttocks ____

18. What is a hamstring?
    a. any of the three muscles of the posterior thigh
    b. flaring cartilaginous expansion on each side of the nare
    c. set of three muscles that run along either side of the spinal column
    d. important muscle for the arm's ability to flex at the elbow ____

19. What is hyperextension?
    a. distribution of nerves in a particular body part
    b. moving a joint to a position beyond its normal limits of extension
    c. point where skeletal muscle is attached to a bone
    d. turning inward, as in turning the soles of the feet toward each other ____

20. What does the term "inferior" mean?
    a. pertaining to the eyelids
    b. back
    c. situated below or lower than a given point of reference
    d. to the side of, or on the side ____

21. What is innervation?
    a. moving a joint to a position beyond its normal limits of extension
    b. transmission of nerve impulses across a synaptic gap
    c. turning inward, as in turning the soles of the feet toward each other
    d. distribution of nerves in a particular body part ____

22. What is the point where skeletal muscle is attached to a bone, skin, or another movable body part?
    a. insertion
    b. origin
    c. abduction
    d. adduction ____

23. Where in the body are intercostal muscles located?
    a. below the knees
    b. between the ribs
    c. between the knuckles
    d. beneath the hips ____

24. What term refers to the middle layer of abdominal muscles?
    a. adductor muscles   c. internal obliques
    b. external obliques   d. arrector pili muscles   ____

25. What term means "turning inward," as in turning the soles of the feet toward each other?
    a. eversion   c. dorsiflexion
    b. rotation   d. insertion   ____

26. What does the term "lateral" mean?
    a. to the side of, or on the side
    b. situated below or lower than a given point of reference
    c. pertaining to the eyelids
    d. back   ____

27. What is a strong fibrous connective tissue that connects bone to bone?
    a. tendon   c. filament
    b. ligament   d. membrane   ____

28. Where in the body is the thick layer of muscle fibers known as the myocardium found?
    a. liver   c. heart
    b. brain   d. stomach   ____

29. What is a special movement of the hand in which the thumb is touched to the fingertips?
    a. dorsiflexion   c. rotation
    b. eversion   d. opposition   ____

30. What term refers to the end point of a muscle that is more fixed (less movable) than the other end point of the muscle?
    a. origin   c. synapse
    b. insertion   d. facia   ____

31. What does the term "palpebral" mean?
    a. to the side of, or on the side
    b. pertaining to the eyelids
    c. situated below or lower than a given point of reference
    d. away from, or farthest from   ____

32. What does the term "posterior" mean?
    a. situated below or lower than a given point of reference
    b. to the side of, or on the side
    c. back
    d. pertaining to the eyelids   ____

33. What term refers to rotation of the forearm that allows the palm to
    face downward or slight inward rotation of the foot while walking?
    a. dorsiflexion   c. adduction
    b. eversion   d. pronation   ____

34. What does the term "proximal" mean?
    a. situated toward the point of origin or attachment
    b. pertaining to the eyelids
    c. situated below or lower than a given point of reference
    d. to the side of, or on the side   ____

35. What does the term "superficial" mean?
    a. to the side of, or on the side
    b. pertaining to the muscles
    c. pertaining to the surface
    d. present in the bloodstream   ____

CHAPTER 6—ANATOMY AND PHYSIOLOGY: THE CARDIOVASCULAR AND LYMPHATIC SYSTEMS

1. What are agranulocytes?
   a. nongranular white blood cells
   b. the smallest branches of veins
   c. contractions of the heart
   d. ions that regulate electric charge   A

2. What is the most abundant blood plasma protein?
   a. atria   c. diastole
   b. albumin   d. systole   B

3. What is the connection point of different parts of a branching network?
   a. pericardium   c. anastomosis
   b. metarteriole   d. basophil   C

4. What is a condition characterized by a deficiency in iron?
   a. arrhythmia   c. thalassemia
   b. cardiomyopathy   d. anemia   D

5. What is the arterial trunk that carries blood from the heart to be distributed by branch arteries through the body?
   a. aorta   c. diastole
   b. systole   d. albumin   A

6. What are the arterioles?
   a. ions that regulate electric charge
   b. the smallest component of the arteries
   c. nongranular white blood cells
   d. connection points of different parts of branching networks   B

7. What term refers to the two upper chambers of the heart that receive blood?
   a. basophil   c. atria
   b. ventricles   d. hypoxia   C

8. What term refers to white blood cells that are characterized by the presence of blue cytoplasmic granules?
   a. agranulocytes   c. aorta
   b. diastole   d. basophils   D

9. What is the force exerted by circulation of the blood on the walls of the blood vessels?
   a. blood pressure
   b. blood friction
   c. blood movement
   d. blood circulation

   A

10. What is part of the normal rhythm of the heart during which the heart chambers fill with blood?
    a. aorta
    b. diastole
    c. agranulocyte
    d. basophil

    B

11. What are ions required by cells to regulate the electric charge and flow of water molecules across the cell membrane?
    a. platelets
    b. agranulocytes
    c. electrolytes
    d. venules

    C

12. What are white blood cells characterized by the presence of cytoplasmic granules that become stained by an acid dye?
    a. basophils
    b. agranulocytes
    c. electrolytes
    d. eosinophils

    D

13. What is the inner layer of the pericardium, which has direct contact with the heart?
    a. epicardium
    b. myocardium
    c. systole
    d. diastole

    A

14. What term refers to red or white blood cells or platelets separated from the fluid part of the blood?
    a. fused elements
    b. formed elements
    c. fused particles
    d. formed particles

    D

15. What term refers to any condition that affects the performance of the heart or the cardiovascular system?
    a. leukemia
    b. heart failure
    c. heart disease
    d. hemophilia

    C

16. What is hyperthermia?
    a. lowering of the body temperature below 95 degrees Fahrenheit
    b. a condition characterized by defective hemoglobin cells
    c. swelling resulting from fluid accumulation
    d. an elevated body temperature

    D

17. What term refers to swelling that commonly occurs in an arm or a leg because of accumulation of interstitial fluids?
    a. anemia
    b. lymphedema
    c. hemophilia
    d. hypoxia

    B

18. What is the region between the lungs, also containing the thymus, esophagus, and trachea and the great vessels?
    a. metarteriole
    b. myocardium
    c. mediastinum
    d. pericardium

    _c_

19. What is a vessel that emerges from an arteriole, passes through the capillary network, and empties into a venule?
    a. mediastinum
    b. pericardium
    c. myocardium
    d. metarteriole

    _D_

20. What is peripheral edema?
    a. swelling resulting from fluid accumulation in the lower limbs
    b. lowering of the body temperature below 95 degrees Fahrenheit
    c. a condition characterized by defective hemoglobin cells
    d. an elevated body temperature

    _A_

21. What are platelets?
    a. the smallest branches of veins
    b. colorless, irregularly shaped components of the blood
    c. the largest branches of arteries
    d. pale yellow transparent fluids that fill body cavities

    _B_

22. What is the path that deoxygenated blood travels to become oxygenated?
    a. pericardium
    b. systemic circulation
    c. pulmonary circulation
    d. epicardium

    _c_

23. What term refers to valves of the arteries that prevent backflow from arteries into the ventricles?
    a. pulmonary
    b. bicuspid
    c. tricuspid
    d. semilunar

    _D_

24. What term describes pale yellow transparent fluids that fill body cavities?
    a. serous
    b. venule
    c. atria
    d. systole

    _A_

25. What is blood and lymph circulation from the heart, through the arteries, to tissues and cells, and back to the heart by way of the veins?
    a. epicardium
    b. systemic circulation
    c. pulmonary circulation
    d. pericardium

    _B_

26. What is hypothermia?
    a. lowering of the body temperature below 95 degrees Fahrenheit
    b. swelling resulting from fluid accumulation
    c. a condition characterized by defective hemoglobin cells
    d. an elevated body temperature   A

27. What is another term for systemic circulation?
    a. normal circulation   c. general circulation
    b. everyday circulation   d. customary circulation   C

28. What does the term "systole" mean?
    a. the part of heart rhythm during which chambers fill with blood
    b. flowing toward the heart
    c. the introduction of oxygen into the bloodstream
    d. contraction of the heart   D

29. What term refers to a weakened pocket of lining in the aorta?
    a. aortic aneurysm   c. aortic hypoxia
    b. aortic failure   d. aortic anemia   A

30. What term refers to inflammation of the pericardium?
    a. pericardium failure
    b. pericarditis
    c. pericardium arrhythmia
    d. pericardium hypoxia   B

31. What is **NOT** a symptom of anemia?
    a. headache
    b. irritability
    c. decreased heart rate
    d. sore or swollen tongue   C

32. What are antibodies?
    a. trace minerals that assist osmotic pressure
    b. chemical messengers that are vital to intercellular
       communication
    c. vitamins that are essential to tissues and organs
    d. proteins dispatched by the immune system to neutralize
       foreign bodies   D

33. What is **NOT** an example of a waste product carried in blood?
    a. albumin   c. urea
    b. lactic acid   d. uric acid   A

34. What are essential to wound healing and tissue continuity?
   a. electrolytes   c. leukocytes
   b. clotting factors   d. respiratory gases   _B_

35. What bodily fluid transports required components to where they are
   needed, while redistributing useless components to where they can be
   properly excreted?
   a. sebum   c. blood
   b. lymph   d. pus   _C_

CHAPTER 7—CHEMISTRY AND BIOCHEMISTRY

1. What term refers to a functional group comprising one nitrogen atom and two hydrogen atoms?
   a. amino group
   b. atomic group
   c. hydrogen group
   d. nitrogen group
   _____

2. What term means "having a painkilling effect"?
   a. aerobic
   b. analgesic
   c. antioxidant
   d. atomic
   _____

3. What is a hydrocarbon containing six carbon atoms and six hydrogen atoms?
   a. amino group
   b. covalent bond
   c. benzene ring structure
   d. carboxyl group
   _____

4. What is a carbon atom double-bonded to an oxygen atom and single-bonded to a hydroxyl group?
   a. covalent bond
   b. amino group
   c. benzene ring structure
   d. carboxyl group
   _____

5. What is an organic compound containing the carboxyl functioning group, a carbon with double-bonded oxygen, and an alcohol group attached?
   a. carboxylic acid
   b. carotenoid
   c. carboxyl group
   d. covalent bond
   _____

6. What are carotenoids?
   a. fatty acids that contain at least one double bond
   b. terpenoid compounds with 40 carbon atoms
   c. lipids made up of multiple isoprene units
   d. vitamins or hormones that assist in an enzyme's activity
   _____

7. What is a stimulant that initiates and/or increases the rate of a chemical reaction?
   a. enzyme
   b. protein
   c. catalyst
   d. element
   _____

8. What is a halogen element, commonly a gas, that is a strong oxidizer with a strong odor?
   a. helium
   b. nitrogen
   c. oxygen
   d. chlorine
   _____

9. What are vitamins or hormones that assist in an enzyme's activity or act as a cofactor?
    a. coenzymes
    b. electrons
    c. flavonoids
    d. flavones

10. What is a covalent bond?
    a. a functional group with one nitrogen atom and two hydrogen atoms
    b. a sharing of electrons between atoms that binds the atoms
    c. an abundant nonmetallic element found in all organic compounds
    d. a reaction between two elements or two compounds

11. What is a sugar made up of two simple sugars such as lactose and sucrose?
    a. flavone
    b. lipid
    c. disaccharide
    d. metabolite

12. What are proteins that regulate and catalyze biological reactions in living organisms?
    a. lipids
    b. carbohydrates
    c. amino acids
    d. enzymes

13. What are electrons?
    a. subatomic particles that carry a negative charge and circle the nucleus
    b. proteins that regulate and catalyze biological reactions
    c. compounds that contain the element carbon
    d. unsaturated fatty acids that contain two or more double bonds

14. What is an equation?
    a. symbol for a particular element on the periodic table
    b. notation representing a chemical reaction
    c. result of fusion between two organic compounds
    d. marking on the side of a test tube containing a pure chemical

15. What is a compound structure that is formed through the reaction of an acid with an alcohol?
    a. fatty wax
    b. fatty acid
    c. ester
    d. lipid

16. What are fatty acids?
    a. hydrocarbon chains with five carbon atoms
    b. lipids made up of multiple isoprene units
    c. subatomic particles found in the nucleus of the atom
    d. lubricant ingredients derived from plant oils or animal fats ____

17. What is an atom or group of atoms that bonds to a reactive area of an organic compound, giving the compound many of its overall characteristics?
    a. functional group   c. carboxyl group
    b. amino group   d. hydroxyl group ____

18. What does the term "hydrophobic" mean?
    a. not absorbing or mixing with oil
    b. not absorbing or mixing with water
    c. easily mixed with oil
    d. easily mixed with water ____

19. What is a bond formed by the attraction between oppositely charged ions?
    a. covalent bond   c. ionic bond
    b. peptide bond   d. fatty bond ____

20. What are isoprene units?
    a. stimulants that increase the rate of chemical reactions
    b. vitamins or hormones that assist in the activity of enzymes
    c. proteins that catalyze biological reactions
    d. hydrocarbon chains with five carbon atoms ____

21. What term refers to a family of carbohydrates made of a single sugar unit that cannot be converted into smaller carbohydrate molecules?
    a. monosaccharide   c. polysaccharide
    b. disaccharide   d. electrosaccharide ____

22. What is the nucleus?
    a. outer shell of the atom
    b. center of the atom
    c. fluid inside the atom's shell
    d. link connecting two atoms ____

23. What are neutrons?
    a. secondary metabolites found in plants
    b. stimulants that increase the rate of chemical reactions
    c. subatomic particles found in the nucleus that carry no charge
    d. hydrocarbon chains with five carbon atoms ____

24. What term refers to compounds that contain the element carbon?
    a. alkaloids
    b. carotenoids
    c. inorganic compounds
    d. organic compounds _____

25. What are peptide bonds?
    a. the primary linkage between all proteins
    b. terpenoid compounds with 40 carbon atoms
    c. vitamins or hormones that assist in the activity of enzymes
    d. proteins that regulate and catalyze biological reactions _____

26. What term refers to a chart of all the known chemical elements, including naturally occurring elements and synthetic elements?
    a. global atlas of the elements
    b. periodic table of the elements
    c. chemical directory of the elements
    d. scientific map of the elements _____

27. What are physiologically active organic compounds containing an aromatic ring and a three-carbon chain?
    a. primary metabolites
    b. polyunsaturated fatty acids
    c. phenylpropanoids
    d. polysaccharides _____

28. What are carbohydrates that contain three or more simple carbohydrate molecules?
    a. disaccharides
    b. monosaccharides
    c. electrosaccharides
    d. polysaccharides _____

29. What term refers to the metabolites required for the growth, structure, and reproduction of a plant?
    a. primary metabolites
    b. key metabolites
    c. essential metabolites
    d. central metabolites _____

30. What are protons?
    a. hydrocarbon chains with five carbon atoms
    b. subatomic particles found in the nucleus that carry a positive charge
    c. stimulants that increase the rate of chemical reactions
    d. secondary metabolites found in plants _____

31. What condition is the result of an oxygen reaction at the unsaturated site of a fatty acid, causing decomposition of the oil and a disagreeable odor?
    a. ionization
    b. rancidity
    c. distillation
    d. alkalinity _____

32. What term refers to fatty acids that contain no double bonds?
    a. polyunsaturated fatty acids   c. saturated fatty acids
    b. secondary fatty acids   d. unsaturated fatty acids   ____

33. What are terpenoid compounds?
    a. electrons in the outermost shell or energy level of the atom
    b. unsaturated fatty acids that contain one double bond in the
       carbon chain
    c. carbohydrates that contain three or more simple carbohydrate
       molecules
    d. lipids made up of multiple isoprene units   ____

34. What are fatty acids that contain at least one double bond?
    a. unsaturated fatty acids
    b. saturated fatty acids
    c. secondary fatty acids
    d. polyunsaturated fatty acids   ____

35. What are valence electrons?
    a. carbohydrates that contain three or more simple carbohydrate
       molecules
    b. electrons in the outermost shell or energy level of the atom
    c. lipids made up of multiple isoprene units
    d. unsaturated fatty acids that contain one double bond in the
       carbon chain   ____

CHAPTER 8—LASER, LIGHT ENERGY, AND RADIOFREQUENCY THERAPY

1. What term refers to the ability to surgically cut or remove using a laser?
   a. ablative
   b. fluence
   c. irradiance
   d. monochromatic

   _H_

2. What term refers to the uptake of one substance into another?
   a. ablation
   b. absorption
   c. maser
   d. lipolysis

   _B_

3. What term refers to the act of removing light energy from a beam before it exits a second medium?
   a. ablation
   b. irradiance
   c. attenuation
   d. fluence

   _C_

4. What is a current that flows on a path of least resistance between positive and negative electrodes that are placed at opposite ends of the treatment forceps or device head?
   a. intense pulsed light (IPL)
   b. microthermal zone (MRT)
   c. optical density (OD)
   d. bipolar radiofrequency (RF) energy

   _D_

5. What term refers to parallel rays of light that travel spatially and temporally in phase with each other?
   a. coherent light
   b. intense pulsed light (IPL)
   c. photomodulation
   d. ultraviolet (UV)

   _A_

6. What is cryogen?
   a. the diameter of the optical or laser light beam
   b. a liquefied gas that is cooled to –238 degrees Fahrenheit
   c. in quantum theory, the elemental unit of light
   d. microwave amplification by stimulated emission of radiation

   _B_

7. What is a "grounding pad" placed on the individual's thigh or an area of large tissue mass that receives the radiofrequency energy?
   a. chromophore
   b. maser
   c. dispersing electrode
   d. optical resonator

   _C_

8. What term refers to irradiance multiplied by the exposure time, measured in joules per square centimeter?
   a. lipolysis
   b. maser
   c. irradiance
   d. fluence

   _D_

9. What is a polychromatic, noncoherent, dispersive band of light commonly using wavelengths from 500 to 1,200 nm?
   a. intense pulsed light (IPL)
   b. coherent light
   c. photomodulation
   d. ultraviolet (UV)

   A

10. What is another term for "power density"?
   a. fluence
   b. irradiance
   c. lipolysis
   d. scatter

   B

11. What are joules?
   a. degrees of heat
   b. measurements of volume
   c. units of energy or work
   d. measurements of weight

   C

12. What are laser-generated air contaminants (LGAC)?
   a. invisible rays that have short wavelengths
   b. hemoglobin in red blood cells that has been oxygenated
   c. a column of tissue that is heated by a fractional laser device
   d. plume of smoke generated from an ablative laser device

   D

13. What term refers to the person responsible for the laser safety program at a facility?
   a. laser safety officer
   b. laser safety deputy
   c. laser protection officer
   d. laser protection deputy

   A

14. What is a device made up of panels of tiny diodes that are pulsed in an exclusive array sequence to trigger a photobiomechanical response?
   a. intense pulsed light (IPL)
   b. light-emitting diode (LED)
   c. coherent light
   d. optical resonator

   B

15. What term refers to the splitting up or destruction of fat cells?
   a. fluence
   b. scatter
   c. lipolysis
   d. irradiance

   C

16. What term refers to the level of laser radiation to which a person may be exposed without hazardous ocular or tissue effects?
   a. nominal hazard zone (NHZ)
   b. optical density (OD)
   c. microthermal zone (MTZ)
   d. maximum permissible exposure (MPE)

   D

17. What term refers to a column of tissue that is heated by a fractional laser device?
   a. microthermal zone (MTZ)
   b. maximum possible exposure (MPE)
   c. nominal hazard zone (NHZ)
   d. optical density (OD)

   A

44

18. What term refers to stimulating or changing cellular function?
    a. scatter
    b. modulate
    c. maser
    d. attenuate

    B

19. What term describes light consisting of one wavelength that is typically found emitted from a laser system?
    a. selective
    b. nominal
    c. monochromatic
    d. thermal

    C

20. What is a deep dermal pigmented lesion usually found on the face in populations of darker-skinned Asians?
    a. joule
    b. microthermal zone (MTZ)
    c. nominal hazard zone (NHZ)
    d. Nevus of Ota

    D

21. What is the zone in which direct, reflected, or scattered radiation, during normal operation, exceeds acceptable limits?
    a. nominal hazard zone (NHZ)
    b. microthermal zone (MTZ)
    c. maximum possible exposure (MPE)
    d. optical density (OD)

    A

22. What term refers to the amount of attenuation or reduction of radiant laser energy as it passes through the filter material in the laser eyewear?
    a. nominal hazard zone (NHZ)
    b. optical density (OD)
    c. microthermal zone (MTZ)
    d. maximum possible exposure (MPE)

    B

23. What term refers to the chronological span of an individual pulse of a laser light?
    a. power density
    b. spot size
    c. pulse duration
    d. scatter

    C

24. What is light-emitting diode (LED) technology that uses energy-producing packets of light to enhance fibroblast collagen synthesis?
    a. cryogen
    b. chromophore
    c. optical resonator
    d. photomodulation

    D

25. What term refers to the rate of energy that is being delivered to tissue by a laser light source?
    a. power density
    b. spot size
    c. scatter
    d. transmission

    A

26. What is another term for "pulse duration"?
    a. pulse size
    b. pulse width
    c. pulse scatter
    d. pulse density

    B

27. What is a treatment using an appropriate wavelength, exposure time, and pulse duration with sufficient energy fluence to absorb light into a specific area?
    a. coherent light
    b. photomodulation
    c. selective photothermolysis
    d. pulse duration

    C

28. What term refers to how long it takes for the target tissue to dissipate one-half of the heat attained by a laser pulse?
    a. microthermal zone (MTZ)
    b. lipolysis
    c. Nevus of Ota
    d. thermal relaxation time (TRT)

    D

29. What is **NOT** true of ultraviolet (UV) rays?
    a. they have long wavelengths
    b. they are invisible
    c. they are the least penetrating rays
    d. they produce chemical effects

    A

30. What is another term for ultraviolet (UV) rays?
    a. hot rays
    b. cold rays
    c. dark rays
    d. bright rays

    B

31. What must the operator do every time a laser treatment is completed?
    a. move the laser device back into a locked storage room
    b. disconnect the laser device from the power source
    c. remove and safely store the control key for the laser
    d. shift the control key to a standby position

    C

32. Who is responsible for regulating firms that manufacture and/or import medical devices sold in America?
    a. Office of Laser Device Oversight (OLDO)
    b. Cosmetic Laser Supervision Department (CLSD)
    c. Radiological Health Esthetic Oversight (RHEO)
    d. Center for Devices and Radiological Health (CDRH)

    D

33. What is **NOT** one of the modes of cooling the skin used during laser treatment?
   a. nominal cooling
   b. precooling
   c. parallel cooling
   d. postcooling

   A

34. What lasers are used primarily for tattoo removal and treatment of pigmented lesions?
   a. erbium glass
   b. photomechanical
   c. pulsed dye layer
   d. Er:YAG

   B

35. Who can verify that a melanin-containing lesion is noncancerous or precancerous?
   a. esthetician
   b. salon manager
   c. physician
   d. laser technician

   C

Part 3: Skin Sciences

CHAPTER 9—WELLNESS MANAGEMENT

1. What term refers to particles created in glycation that cross-link with proteins and lipids, resulting in tissue damage?
   a. AGE products
   b. antioxidants
   c. free radicals
   d. neurotransmitters
   ____

2. What is the part of the metabolic process during which larger molecules are built up from smaller molecules?
   a. glycation
   b. anabolism
   c. catabolism
   d. Maillard reaction
   ____

3. What are substances that neutralize free radicals?
   a. cortisol and adrenaline
   b. AGE products
   c. antioxidants
   d. neurotransmitters
   ____

4. What can create a state of agitation?
   a. caffeine
   b. fats
   c. salt
   d. sugar
   ____

5. What indicates a deficiency of vitamin A?
   a. brittle hair and nails
   b. excessive oiliness
   c. skin infections and mouth sores
   d. dermatitis
   ____

6. What is the part of the metabolic process during which larger molecules within cells are broken down into smaller molecules?
   a. Maillard reaction
   b. glycation
   c. anabolism
   d. catabolism
   ____

7. How many calories are there in one gram of fat?
   a. three
   b. five
   c. seven
   d. nine
   ____

8. What is a hormone that allows the body to address a threatening situation by releasing energy from fat cells for use in the muscles?
   a. cortisol
   b. adrenaline
   c. calcium
   d. magnesium
   ____

9. What indicates a deficiency of riboflavin?
   a. dermatitis
   b. excessive oiliness
   c. brittle hair and nails
   d. skin infections and mouth sores   ____

10. What can cause sluggishness?
    a. caffeine   c. salt
    b. fats   d. sugar   ____

11. What organ stimulates the fight-or-flight response, which prepares
    the body for trauma?
    a. heart   c. stomach
    b. brain   d. liver   ____

12. What are free radicals?
    a. hormones that elevate the heart rate and increase blood pressure
    b. hormones that allow the body to address threatening situations
    c. unstable molecules that have broken away from weak molecules
    d. chemical messengers synthesized from food   ____

13. What is the chemical reaction produced by browning foods or
    cooking them at high temperatures, thereby creating AGE products?
    a. anabolism   c. catabolism
    b. glycation   d. Maillard reaction   ____

14. How many calories are there in one gram of carbohydrate?
    a. two   c. six
    b. four   d. eight   ____

15. What are substances that travel across synapses to act on or inhibit a
    target cell?
    a. neurotransmitters   c. external triggers
    b. free radicals   d. internal triggers   ____

16. What varies by body height and the level of physical activity?
    a. value of carbohydrates
    b. amount of calories needed
    c. value of fats
    d. importance of a healthy diet   ____

17. What indicates a deficiency of niacin?
    a. dermatitis
    b. brittle hair and nails
    c. skin infections and mouth sores
    d. excessive oiliness   _____

18. What can cause dehydration and increased water retention?
    a. caffeine   c. salt
    b. fats   d. sugar   _____

19. How many calories are there in one gram of protein?
    a. two   c. six
    b. four   d. eight   _____

20. What happens when people who are aging eat the same amount of
    food they always have without increasing the amount of exercise?
    a. weight gain   c. diabetes
    b. hair loss   d. high blood pressure   _____

21. What happens to metabolism as a person ages?
    a. speeds up   c. fluctuates greatly
    b. slows down   d. ceases altogether   _____

22. What foods are **NOT** excellent antioxidants?
    a. nuts   c. red meats
    b. leafy green vegetables   d. whole grains   _____

23. What is **NOT** a negative effect of consuming too much sugar?
    a. depleting the body of B vitamins, which help moderate stress
    b. allowing an overgrowth of yeast cells in the body
    c. throwing the digestive system off-balance
    d. stimulating an unhealthy amount of weight loss   _____

24. What indicates a deficiency of pyridoxine?
    a. excessive oiliness
    b. skin infections and mouth sores
    c. brittle hair and nails
    d. dermatitis   _____

25. How many energy calories are contained in one food calorie?
    a. 10   c. 1,000
    b. 100   d. 10,000   _____

26. Why do the types of food ingested have a large effect on neurotransmitters' behavior?
    a. neurotransmitters are synthesized from nutrients in food
    b. the body can only synthesize neurotransmitters from sugar
    c. salty foods destroy the body's natural neurotransmitters
    d. food ingestion has no effect on neurotransmitters' behavior _____

27. What does a lack of seratonin cause?
    a. acne breakout   c. bloating
    b. bad mood   d. cold sweat _____

28. Why do high-carbohydrate foods such as pastries provide a calming effect?
    a. they actually cause a stressful effect
    b. these foods normalize blood pressure
    c. they facilitate seratonin production
    d. these foods normalize digestion _____

29. What is one way to manage either food sensitivities or allergies?
    a. eat only fruits and vegetables
    b. build meals from tiny portions of many different foods
    c. buy supplements that promise to boost your immune system
    d. write down everything you eat for a certain time period _____

30. What can lead to anxiety, fatigue, headaches, and irritability?
    a. caffeine   c. salt
    b. fats   d. sugar _____

31. What is great to do before you enter what you know will be a stressful situation?
    a. take slow, deep cleansing breaths
    b. consume a large amount of caffeine
    c. eat a heavy pasta dish
    d. exercise to raise your heart rate _____

32. What does it mean to "put on the brakes" when facing a stressful situation?
    a. halt the situation to consume a helpful jolt of caffeine
    b. slow down your breathing, movements, and speech
    c. take your mind off the situation and think about a favorite food
    d. raise your voice so others cannot speak over you _____

33. What is the first part of the body that the brain alerts upon encountering a threat?
    a. pituitary gland   c. hypothalamus
    b. adrenal glands   d. fat cells   ____

34. What is a negative effect of using cigarettes to control eating?
    a. the smoker avoids excess calories
    b. snacking between meals decreases
    c. fewer "second helpings" are eaten
    d. the skin is malnourished   ____

35. How much more AGE product content does a fried egg have than a hard-boiled egg?
    a. 100 times more   c. 10,000 times more
    b. 1,000 times more   d. 100,000 times more   ____

CHAPTER 10—ADVANCED SKIN DISORDERS: SKIN IN DISTRESS

1. What term refers to pink, sometimes scaly, abnormal skin lesions that are considered precancerous?
   a. actinic keratosis
   b. cytokine
   c. chalazia
   d. retention hyperkeratosis

   A

2. What term refers to certain cosmetics and skin care products that contain fats, fatty derivatives, or waxes that are known to cause or worsen development of acne?
   a. dysplastic
   b. papulopustular
   c. erythematotelangiectatic
   d. comedogenic

   D

3. What is a molecule secreted by an activated or stimulated cell that causes chemical immune responses in certain other cells?
   a. actinic keratosis
   b. chalazia
   c. cytokine
   d. retention hyperkeratosis

   C

4. What is *demodex folliculorium*?
   a. a form of male hormone that stimulates the sebaceous glands
   b. sudden facial redness caused by blood rushing to the skin
   c. fluid oozing from a healing wound
   d. a skin mite that has been associated with rosacea

   D

5. What is dihydrotestosterone (DHT)?
   a. a form of male hormone that stimulates the sebaceous glands
   b. a skin mite that has been associated with rosacea
   c. sudden facial redness caused by blood rushing to the skin
   d. fluid oozing from a healing wound

   A

6. What is a subtype of rosacea that often resembles acne vulgaris, with large red pustules and papules?
   a. granulomatous rosacea
   b. ocular rosacea
   c. erythematotelangiectatic rosacea
   d. papulopustular rosacea

   D

7. What term means "relating to abnormal growth"?
   a. comedogenic
   b. dysplastic
   c. erythematotelangiectatic
   d. papulopustular

   B

8. What term refers to a subtype of rosacea that is characterized by diffuse, patchy redness and a grainy texture?
   a. dysplastic
   b. comedogenic
   c. erythematotelangiectatic
   d. papulopustular rosacea

   c

9. What are exudates?
   a. male hormones that stimulate the sebaceous glands
   b. skin mites that have been associated with rosacea
   c. episodes of sudden facial redness caused by blood rushing to the skin
   d. fluids oozing from healing wounds

   D

10. What is an ostium?
    a. the bacterium that causes acne vulgaris
    b. a splotchy freckling of hyperpigmentation
    c. the opening of a follicle on the skin surface
    d. a type of yeast associated with seborrheic dermatitis

    C

11. What term refers to an episode in which pimples and redness occur in a person who has rosacea?
    a. flare
    b. trigger
    c. chloasma
    d. melasma

    A

12. What term refers to sudden facial redness caused by blood rushing to the skin?
    a. chloasma
    b. flushing
    c. hemostasis
    d. reepithelialization

    B

13. What is granulomatous rosacea?
    a. a skin mite that has been associated with rosacea
    b. sudden facial redness caused by blood rushing to the skin
    c. any form of rosacea that includes hard, nodular papules
    d. a type of intestinal bacterium that has been associated with rosacea

    C

14. What is reepithelialization?
    a. redness that comes and goes
    b. the formation of new epidermis and dermis over an area of injury
    c. an acnelike condition around the mouth
    d. the phase of wound healing with increased vascularity

    B

15. What term refers to crusty-looking, slightly raised lesions in mature, sun-damaged skin?
    a. basal cell carcinoma
    c. seborrheic keratoses
    b. squamous cell carcinoma
    d. rhinophyma

    _C_

16. What is mottling?
    a. splotchy freckling of hyperpigmentation
    b. opening of a follicle on the skin service
    c. bacterium that causes acne vulgaris
    d. arrest or control of bleeding

    _A_

17. What is *helicobacter pylori*?
    a. sudden facial redness caused by blood rushing to the skin
    b. a skin mite that has been associated with rosacea
    c. any form of rosacea that includes hard, nodular papules
    d. a type of intestinal bacterium that has been associated with rosacea

    _D_

18. What is hemostasis?
    a. the arrest or control of bleeding
    b. a splotchy freckling of hyperpigmentation
    c. the opening of a follicle on the skin surface
    d. the bacterium that causes acne vulgaris

    _A_

19. What are hordeolums?
    a. inflamed pustules
    c. clogged follicles
    b. infected tear ducts
    d. ingrown hairs

    _B_

20. What term refers to inflammation that can be seen with the naked eye or with the aid of a magnifying loupe?
    a. reepithelialization
    c. clinical inflammation
    b. inflammation cascade
    d. cross-linking

    _C_

21. What are also called "styes"?
    a. chalazia
    c. hordeolums
    b. exudates
    d. ostiums

    _C_

22. What are enzymes that break down substances in the skin and are produced by the skin when it is inflamed?
    a. demodex folliculorium
    b. helicobacter pylori
    c. pityrosporum ovale
    d. matrix metalloproteinases

    _D_

23. What is a subtype of rosacea that affects the eyes, resulting in eye redness, swollen eyelids, and other eye lesions?
    a. granulomatous rosacea
    b. ocular rosacea
    c. erythematotelangiectatic rosacea
    d. papulopustular rosacea

    B

24. What is a process in which collagen and elastin fibrils in the dermis collapse, causing the support system for the skin to collapse?
    a. cross-linking   c. inflammation cascade
    b. reepithelialization   d. clinical inflammation

    A

25. What term refers to small, lumpy cysts in the eyelids?
    a. retention hyperkeratosis   c. actinic keratosis
    b. chalazia   d. cytokine

    B

26. What is transient erythema?
    a. the formation of new epidermis and dermis over an area of injury
    b. redness that comes and goes
    c. the phase of wound healing with increased vascularity
    d. an acnelike condition around the mouth

    B

27. What is cryotherapy?
    a. a form of male hormone that stimulates the sebaceous glands
    b. dermatological removal of lesions by freezing
    c. the body's delivery of white blood cells to inflammation sites
    d. using a lancet to open a follicle on the skin surface

    B

28. What is perioral dermatitis?
    a. an acnelike condition around the mouth
    b. sudden facial redness caused by blood rushing to the skin
    c. a splotchy freckling of hyperpigmentation
    d. a type of yeast associated with seborrheic dermatitis

    A

29. What is *pityrosporum ovale*?
    a. an acnelike condition around the mouth
    b. a type of yeast associated with seborrheic dermatitis
    c. sudden facial redness caused by blood rushing to the skin
    d. a splotchy freckling of hyperpigmentation

    B

30. What is postinflammatory hyperpigmentation?
    a. sudden facial redness caused by blood rushing to the skin
    b. the formation of new epidermis and dermis over an area
       of injury
    c. dark melanin splotches caused by trauma to the skin
    d. a subtype of rosacea that resembles acne vulgaris   *c*

31. What term refers to the phase of wound healing in which there is
    increased vascularity to supply nutrients and oxygen to the wound?
    a. remodeling   c. cytokine
    b. dysplastic   d. proliferative   *D*

32. What is *propionibacterium acnes?*
    a. the bacterium that causes acne vulgaris
    b. a type of yeast associated with seborrheic dermatitis
    c. a splotchy freckling of hyperpigmentation
    d. sudden facial redness caused by blood rushing to the skin *A*

33. What term refers to the maturation phase of a wound?
    a. dysplastic   c. remodeling
    b. proliferative   d. cytokine   *c*

34. What term refers to a hereditary condition in which dead skin cells
    are kept rather than shed?
    a. actinic keratosis   c. melasma
    b. chloasma   d. retention hyperkeratosis   *D*

35. What term refers to enlarging of the nose resulting from a severe
    form of acne rosacea?
    a. rhinophyma   c. reepithelialization
    b. squamous cell carcinoma d. basal cell carcinoma   *A*

CHAPTER 11—SKIN TYPING AND AGING ANALYSIS

1. When should you take notes about client response to treatment and home care?
   a. only on the first visit
   b. once per year
   c. twice per year
   d. each time you see the client

   D

2. What are you prepared to do once you have recorded skin-analysis information on a client assessment form?
   a. create a treatment plan and home care regimen
   b. prescribe skin care medication
   c. guarantee permanent improvement of the clients' skin
   d. recommend cosmetic surgery

   A

3. What ethnic background is rated "1" on the Lancer Ethnicity Scale?
   a. Nordic, Celtic (Irish, Scottish)
   b. Native American Indian
   c. Chinese, Japanese, Korean
   d. Central/East/West African

   A

4. How can a client help improve the quality of his or her skin and achieve a higher level of satisfaction regarding his or her skin care?
   a. use only the most expensive skin care products on the market
   b. change behaviors that affect the skin, such as sun exposure
   c. get corrective surgery even if no skin problems are evident
   d. purchase professional skin care machines for home use

   B

5. What does the Fitzpatrick typing method measure?
   a. amount of photodamage the skin has suffered
   b. ethnicity and geographic origin of the client's skin
   c. amount of pigment in the skin and its tolerance to the sun
   d. androgen/estrogen balance of the client's body

   C

6. What is the most important information that Fitzpatrick skin typing provides?
   a. how the skin will respond to treatment
   b. how long the client will live
   c. what products will aggravate a client's allergies
   d. what diseases the client will have

   A

7. What ethnic background is rated "2" on the Lancer Ethnicity Scale?
   a. Nordic, Celtic (Irish, Scottish)
   b. Central/Eastern European
   c. Thai, Vietnamese
   d. Arabic, North African, Middle East

   B

8. How many Fitzpatrick skin types are there?
   a. two   c. six
   b. four   d. eight

   C

9. What is fairer skin more likely to display because capillaries show through its translucent layer?
   a. hyperpigmentation   c. hypopigmentation
   b. visible redness   d. acne vulgaris

   B

10. How does darker skin typically respond to trauma?
    a. hypopigmentation   c. acne vulgaris
    b. visible redness   d. hyperpigmentation

    D

11. What Fitzpatrick skin types are likely to have a quick response and possibly deeper treatment?
    a. types I–III   c. types III and IV
    b. types IV–VI   d. types II and VI

    A

12. What ethnic background is rated "3" on the Lancer Ethnicity Scale?
    a. Northern European   c. Native American Indian
    b. Central/Eastern European d. Entrian and Ethiopian

    C

13. What Fitzpatrick skin types may be difficult to treat and have troubling complications such as hyperpigmentation and hypopigmentation?
    a. types I–III   c. types II and IV
    b. types IV–VI   d. types II and VI

    B

14. What element of Fitzpatrick skin typing indicates the propensity of a given skin to react in a predictable manner to a given treatment?
    a. hair color   c. skin coloration
    b. eye color   d. reaction to sun

    C

15. What question is found in the Genetic Disposition part of the Fitzpatrick Identification Form?
    a. What happens when you stay too long in the sun?
    b. When did you last expose your body to the sun?
    c. To what degree do you turn brown?
    d. What is the natural color of your hair?

    D

16. What question is found in the Reaction to Sun Exposure part of the Fitzpatrick Identification Form?
    a. To what degree do you turn brown?
    b. Do you have freckles on unexposed areas?
    c. What color are your eyes?
    d. What is the natural color of your hair?

    A

17. What ethnic background is rated "4" on the Lancer Ethnicity Scale?
    a. Northern European
    b. Native American Indian
    c. Ashkenazi Jewish
    d. Filipino, Polynesian

    D

18. What should the esthetician consider when conducting skin typing for peels or treatments that may require healing?
    a. the fact that skin types around the world are all the same
    b. the unprecedented integration and mixing of ethnicities
    c. the fact that peels are legally banned for older clients
    d. gender and age are the only considerations for peels

    B

19. When was the Roberts Skin Type Classification System developed?
    a. 1888
    b. 1928
    c. 1978
    d. 2008

    D

20. What does the term "*i/i/i*" stand for?
    a. infection, infirmary, and impact
    b. integumentary/interior/infection
    c. inflammation, injury, and insult
    d. irradiation/inflammation/infection

    C

21. What ethnic background is rated "5" on the Lancer Ethnicity Scale?
    a. Central/East/West African
    b. Ashkenazi Jewish
    c. Central/Eastern European
    d. Northern European

    A

22. What is the esthetician trying to determine by asking a client what color the client's skin turns during a breakout or a cut?
    a. presence of cancerous tissue
    b. postinflammatory hyperpigmentation
    c. presence of contagious disease
    d. degree of photodamage

    B

23. Where on the client's body is a test patch done to determine any possible pigment problems?
    a. back
    b. chest
    c. near the ear
    d. near the navel

    c

24. What is the benefit of using skin typing systems, in addition to determining skin type?
    a. guaranteeing treatment results
    b. diagnosing internal diseases
    c. adding a charge to the client's bill
    d. setting realistic expectations

    D

25. What helps create a positive relationship and improve awareness of potential outcome?
    a. communication   c. retail sales
    b. home care   d. massage treatments

    A

26. What is typically considered the gold standard in skin typing today?
    a. Bauman Skin Type Solution
    b. Fitzpatrick skin typing
    c. Willis and Earles Scale
    d. Taylor Hyperpigmentation Scale

    B

27. What skin typing system might you combine with the Fitzpatrick method if your practice has mainly African American clients?
    a. Goldman World Classification
    b. The Lancer System
    c. Kawada Skin Classification System
    d. Willis and Earles Scale

    D

28. What is the Lancer system commonly combined with the Fitzpatrick method to do?
    a. shorten the skin analysis
    b. diagnose internal disease
    c. achieve an accurate skin type
    d. reduce treatment costs

    C

29. What term refers to aging that is the result of genetics?
    a. intrinsic   c. estrogen
    b. androgen   d. extrinsic

    A

30. What term refers to aging that is the result of exposure to environmental conditions such as pollution, solar damage, or even cigarette smoke?
    a. estrogen   c. intrinsic
    b. extrinsic   d. androgen

    B

31. When was the Glogau scale developed?
    a. 1890s   c. 1960s
    b. 1930s   d. 1990s

    D

32. What system helps physicians standardize their approach in addressing problems and communicate with each other about a client's issues?
    a. Lancer System
    b. Willis and Earles Scale
    c. Glogau scale
    d. Kawada System

    C

33. What is the Glogau scale based upon?
    a. visual assessment
    b. patch tests
    c. blood samples
    d. cellular analysis

    A

34. What is true about the incorporation of acne scarring and the use of makeup into Glogau system evaluations of the skin?
    a. incorporating these elements makes the system simpler than others
    b. incorporating these elements is a confusing aspect of the system
    c. neither of these elements is incorporated into the system
    d. only acne scarring, and not makeup, is incorporated into the system

    B

35. How many classifications of photodamage are there in the Glogau scale?
    a. two
    b. four
    c. six
    d. eight

    B

CHAPTER 12—SKIN CARE PRODUCTS: CHEMISTRY, INGREDIENTS, AND SELECTION

1. What term refers to a family of plant-based antioxidants, most often found in the leaves of the tea plant?
   - a. catechins
   - b. retinoids
   - c. polyphenols
   - d. free acids

   A

2. What is esterification?
   - a. process of losing esters
   - b. process of creating an ester
   - c. penetration of an ester into skin
   - d. discharge of an ester from skin

   B

3. What term refers to acid molecules that have not been neutralized?
   - a. glycolic acid
   - b. mandelic acid
   - c. free acid
   - d. lactic acid

   C

4. What is the smallest of the alpha hydroxy acids (AHAs)?
   - a. mandelic acid
   - b. salicylic acid
   - c. free acid
   - d. gylcolic acid

   D

5. What does the term "in vitro" mean?
   - a. in the laboratory
   - b. in a living organism
   - c. not yet neutralized
   - d. not yet polymerized

   A

6. What does the term "in vivo" mean?
   - a. in the laboratory
   - b. in a living organism
   - c. not yet polymerized
   - d. not yet neutralized

   B

7. What is the second smallest of the AHAs?
   - a. free acid
   - b. gylcolic acid
   - c. lactic acid
   - d. mandelic acid

   C

8. What term refers to energy from the sun that travels through space in the form of visible light?
   - a. light amplification
   - b. light transmission
   - c. light radiation
   - d. light iridescence

   C

9. What is the result of a chemical process that brings a formulation's pH to 7.0?
   - a. polymerization
   - b. esterification
   - c. light radiation
   - d. neutralization

   D

10. What pH measurement represents a neutral pH?
    a. 3.0   c. 7.0
    b. 5.0   d. 9.0   C

11. What term refers to ingredients derived from an agricultural product
    that has been processed under the guidelines of the USDA's Natural
    Organic Program?
    a. organic ingredients   c. agricultural ingredients   A
    b. natural ingredients   d. homegrown ingredients

12. What is polymerization?
    a. process of losing polymers
    b. process of creating a polymer
    c. penetration of polymer into skin
    d. discharge of polymer from skin   B

13. What are polyphenols?
    a. vitamin A derivatives
    b. the smallest of the AHAs
    c. plant-based antioxidants
    d. a group of chemicals that act as antioxidants   D

14. What vitamin are retinoids derived from?
    a. vitamin A   c. vitamin C
    b. vitamin B   d. vitamin D   A

15. What is rentinyl palmitate?
    a. vitamin D derivative   c. light energy from the sun
    b. mild retinoid   d. neutralized acid molecule   B

16. What term refers to the science of formulating and producing the
    products used in the esthetics profession and by consumers at home?
    a. cosmetic production   c. cosmetic chemistry   C
    b. esthetic production   d. esthetic chemistry

17. What is **NOT** produced by cosmetic chemists?
    a. cleansers   c. foundation makeup
    b. moisturizers   d. essential oils   D

18. What is the study of how drugs and chemicals affect the body's
    function?
    a. pharmacology   c. chemistry
    b. biology   d. cosmetology   A

19. What term refers to the ingredients that provide the greatest benefit to the skin and give cosmetic products their treatment value?
    a. functional ingredients   c. natural ingredients
    b. performance ingredients   d. organic ingredients   *B*

20. What must the esthetician have in order to keep up with new ingredients, new products, and new technologies?
    a. broad knowledge of advanced chemistry concepts
    b. extensive laboratory experience
    c. general understanding of what already exists
    d. extensive scientific training   *C*

21. Why do clients tend to want immediate results from professional skin care?
    a. actually, most clients understand that skin care takes time
    b. clients only seek professional help shortly before special events
    c. most skin care clients are suffering from serious skin diseases
    d. they tend to seek solutions once problems are already evident   *D*

22. What are sometimes referred to as "active principles"?
    a. performance ingredients   c. natural ingredients
    b. functional ingredients   d. organic ingredients   *A*

23. What term refers to a specific chemical component of a botanical?
    a. formulator   c. emulsifier
    b. fraction   d. emollient   *B*

24. What are occasionally called "carriers"?
    a. botanicals   c. vehicles
    b. chemicals   d. fractions   *C*

25. What products are especially susceptible to developing bacteria, fungus, and mold unless preservatives are added to the products?
    a. oil-based products
    b. water-based products
    c. chemically formulated products
    d. products that contain plant extracts   *D*

26. What is **NOT** true of an ideal preservative system?
    a. narrow antibacterial spectrum   c. nonirritating
    b. compatible with other ingredients d. nonsensitizing   *A*

27. What is **NOT** an example of a certification-exempt color?
    a. annatto extract   c. beta-carotene
    b. inorganic pigment   d. copper powder   *B*

28. What is absent from a product that is marked "hypoallergenic"?
    a. moisture
    b. spreadability
    c. fragrance
    d. density

    C

29. What is an ingredient's first barrier to penetration of the skin?
    a. stratum granulosum
    b. stratum lucidum
    c. stratum spinosum
    d. stratum corneum

    D

30. What is the second obstacle to product penetration?
    a. epidermal-dermal junction
    b. stratum spinosum
    c. stratum granulosum
    d. epidermis

    A

31. What term refers to the location where performance ingredients take action?
    a. impact zone
    b. target site
    c. action area
    d. performance place

    B

32. When were AHAs introduced in skin care cosmetics?
    a. 1940s
    b. 1960s
    c. 1980s
    d. 2000s

    C

33. What is **NOT** an example of an AHA?
    a. lactic acid
    b. malic acid
    c. tartaric acid
    d. salicylic acid

    D

34. What is a broad-based term encompassing the techniques, materials, and instruments that function at the scale of one-millionth of a millimeter?
    a. nanotechnology
    b. biochemistry
    c. microbiology
    d. atomic science

    A

35. What prevents hyaluronic acid from penetrating the skin?
    a. high oil content
    b. large molecular size
    c. low water content
    d. chemical instability

    B

CHAPTER 13—BOTANICALS AND AROMATHERAPY

1. What is an extraction method using a solvent (hexane) to extract the essence from the plant material?
   a. absolute
   b. adulteration
   c. olfaction
   d. synergy

   A

2. What is the process of adding natural or synthetic compounds, or cheaper but similar oils, to "stretch" or alter the fragrance of an essential oil?
   a. tincture
   b. adulteration
   c. absolute
   d. infusion

   B

3. What is an anti-inflammatory compound isolated from the herb comfrey?
   a. helichrysum
   b. shea butter
   c. allantoin
   d. arnica

   C

4. What chemical family includes needle tree oils such as cypress, pine, and spruce?
   a. sesquiterpene hydrocarbons
   b. monoterpene hydrocarbons
   c. aldehydes
   d. esters

   B

5. What is used in skin-soothing cosmetics for its ability to heal wounds and skin ulcers and to stimulate the growth of healthy tissue?
   a. arnica
   b. helichrysum
   c. shea butter
   d. allantoin

   D

6. What is an antioxidant nutrient used in skin care and health supplements, generally isolated from soy or wheat?
   a. alpha D-tocopherol
   b. hydrosol
   c. DL-tocopherol
   d. supercritical carbon dioxide

   A

7. What vitamin is alpha D-tocopherol a form of?
   a. vitamin A
   b. vitamin C
   c. vitamin E
   d. vitamin K

   C

8. What chemical family includes German chamomile?
   a. esters
   b. monoterpene hydrocarbons
   c. sesquiterpene hydrocarbons
   d. aldehydes

   C

9. What is an aqueous extract?
   a. nonvolatile fatty oil derived from vegetables and fruits
   b. herbal water infusion
   c. anti-inflammatory compound isolated from the herb comfrey
   d. volatile fatty oil

   B

10. How is the botanical arnica available?
    a. in a butter form
    b. as a powdered extract and tincture
    c. as a dried herb or infusion
    d. as a whole juice or powder

    c

11. What is the amount, usually defined as a percentage, to which essential oils are adulterated in a formula when added to a cream, oil, or perfume blend?
    a. adulteration amount   c. fixed amount
    b. absolute amount   d. dilution amount

    D

12. What is distillation?
    a. process that removes mineral and trace elements from water
    b. use of a solvent to extract essence from plant material
    c. placing a plant material in a high-pressure container with CO_2
    d. using alcohol or glycerin to extract compounds from plant material

    A

13. What chemical family includes lemon verberna, lemongrass, and citronella?
    a. esters
    b. sesquiterpene hydrocarbons
    c. monoterpene hydrocarbons
    d. aldehydes

    D

14. What is a synthetic form of vitamin E?
    a. supercritical carbon dioxide
    b. DL-tocopherol
    c. alpha D-tocopherol
    d. hydrosol

    B

15. What is a fixed oil?
    a. water portion of essential oil distillation
    b. synthetic form of vitamin E
    c. nonvolatile fatty oil derived from vegetables and fruits
    d. herbal water infusion

    c

16. What is a definition and standard developed several years ago by
    French insurance companies to label the essential oils suitable for
    patient reimbursement?
    a. natural and handmade   c. original and therapeutic
    b. certified and organic   d. genuine and authentic   _D_

17. What term refers to the philosophy or practice that sees the body as a
    whole?
    a. holistic health   c. total care
    b. whole-body wellness   d. organic healing   _A_

18. What chemical family includes lavender, bergamot, and chamomile?
    a. esters
    b. aldehydes
    c. monoterpene hydrocarbons
    d. sesquiterpene hydrocarbons   _A_

19. How is the botanical aloe vera available?
    a. dried herb or infusion
    b. whole juice or powder
    c. powdered extract and tincture
    d. butter form   _B_

20. What is **NOT** one of the considerations that comprises the concept
    of holistic health?
    a. emotions   c. lifestyle
    b. artistic talent   d. environment   _B_

21. What is the water portion, or by-product, of essential oil distillation?
    a. allantoin   c. hydrosol
    b. DL-tocopherol   d. alpha D-tocopherol   _C_

22. What does the term "nonvolatile" mean?
    a. immiscible with water   c. does not liquefy easily
    b. immiscible with oil   d. does not evaporate easily   _D_

23. What chemical family includes clove and cinnamon?
    a. phenols   c. lactones
    b. phenylpropanes   d. oxide   _B_

24. What term describes the result of redistilling essential oils to remove
    color and unwanted compounds from the oil?
    a. rectified   c. refined
    b. adulterated   d. infused   _A_

25. What term describes a plant extract, usually referring to a fixed oil, that has gone through the process of removing colors, odors, or other naturally occurring compounds?
    a. infused
    b. refined
    c. rectified
    d. adulterated

    B

26. What is a modern method of extraction in which the plant material is placed in a high-pressure container with an element midway between its gaseous and liquid states?
    a. hydrosol
    b. alpha D-tocopherol
    c. supercritical carbon dioxide
    d. DL-tocopherol

    C

27. What chemical family includes oregano, savory, and thyme thymol?
    a. oxide
    b. phenylpropanes
    c. phenols
    d. lactones

    C

28. What term refers to extracts from plant materials that have not been changed or altered from their extracted form?
    a. absolute
    b. aqueous extract
    c. herbal infusion
    d. whole extract

    D

29. What is **NOT** part of the chemical structure of the botanical arnica?
    a. silica
    b. alkaloids
    c. flavonoids
    d. tannins

    A

30. What chemical family includes eucalyptus oils, tea tree, and ravensare?
    a. lactones
    b. phenols
    c. phenylpropanes
    d. oxide

    D

31. How is the botanical bamboo available?
    a. whole juice or powder
    b. butter form
    c. dried herb or infusion
    d. powdered extract and tincture

    D

32. How is the botanical cocoa available?
    a. butter or powder
    b. powdered extract and tincture
    c. dried herb or infusion
    d. whole juice or powder

    A

33. What chemical family includes *graveolens* and *inula*?
    a. lactones
    b. phenylpropanes
    c. phenols
    d. oxides

    A

34. What essential oil features atlantone-7 (a mild keratone) and cedrol (a sesquiterpene alcohol) as its main components?
    a. chamomile
    b. cedarwood
    c. eucalyptus
    d. geranium

    B

35. What essential oil features aldehydes, cineole (oxide), and monoterpene alcohols as its main components?
    a. geranium
    b. cedarwood
    c. eucalyptus
    d. chamomile

    C

CHAPTER 14—INGREDIENTS AND PRODUCTS FOR SKIN ISSUES

1. What is the most important factor in recommending the right home care for your clients?
   a. skin analysis
   b. chemical ingredients
   c. natural ingredients
   d. product labeling

   A

2. What is an important step in the process of recommending products for clients?
   a. learning how to formulate cosmetic chemicals
   b. being able to read and decipher cosmetic labels
   c. learning how to extract properties from plant materials
   d. being able to sell clients products they do not really need

   B

3. What is essential to understanding product cost?
   a. there is no need for you to understand product cost
   b. you are only expected to understand your salon's profit margin
   c. understanding how a product is developed
   d. understanding how much other salons are charging for the product

   C

4. What do estheticians often find to be the only cosmetic product that clients regularly use?
   a. creams
   b. ampoules
   c. masks
   d. cleansers

   D

5. What does **NOT** affect how a cleanser functions or might make it more appropriate for a specific skin type and condition?
   a. whether it foams
   b. presence of moisturizing ingredients
   c. whether it dries the skin
   d. presence of correcting ingredients

   A

6. What is **NOT** one of the normal means of removing cleanser from the face?
   a. wiping with moistened cotton pads
   b. wiping with a dry paper towel
   c. rinsing with water
   d. removing with toner

   B

7. Why should you use filtered water to rinse off cleanser if the tap water in your salon is very alkaline ("hard" water)?
   a. hard water is usually very dirty
   b. filtered water has natural cleansers
   c. hard water can be drying
   d. filtered water smoothes the skin

   C

8. What is **NOT** true about cleansers that contain alpha hydroxy acids (AHAs) and beta hydroxy acids (BHAs)?
   a. they gently exfoliate as they cleanse
   b. they often contain soothing botanicals
   c. they do not need to be followed up with a toner
   d. they have a pH of 7.5 or higher

   D

9. What is true about products that are labeled "astringents"?
   a. they are considered to be over-the-counter (OTC) drugs
   b. they occlude the skin
   c. they can only be administered in a medical office
   d. they are not approved for direct application to the skin

   A

10. What products help to temporarily shrink the appearance of pore size?
    a. cleansers   c. creams
    b. toners   d. moisturizers

    B

11. What is often the basis for the distinction between each subclassification of creams?
    a. type of packaging in which particular creams are sold
    b. demographic to which specific creams are marketed
    c. type of ingredients incorporated into the formulation
    d. price is the only significant reason for subclassifications

    C

12. Why are milder ingredients usually used for eye and neck creams?
    a. this guarantees brief shelf life, which in turn stimulates repeat purchases
    b. this allows interaction with makeup
    c. skin in those areas ages very slowly and requires little care
    d. skin in those areas may be sensitive

    D

13. What is one of the reasons that night creams tend to have nourishing or performance ingredients?
    a. it is believed the body absorbs these ingredients better while resting
    b. these ingredients have odors that would be unacceptable during the day
    c. these ingredients are incompatible with makeup
    d. it is not true that night creams have these ingredients

    A

14. What ingredient might a performance cream contain for hyperpigmentation?
    a. tea tree oil
    b. kojic acid
    c. hydrogen peroxide
    d. benzoyl peroxide

    B

15. Why are antioxidants an important consideration for products targeting hyperpigmentation?
    a. products targeting this condition cannot contain antioxidants
    b. hyperpigmentation is stimulated by antioxidants
    c. pigment formation is an oxidation-mediated reaction
    d. a product with antioxidants will immediately correct this condition

    C

16. What is it recommended to stress when recommending performance creams that are AHA- or BHA-based?
    a. regular exfoliation
    b. nightly cleansing
    c. light use of makeup
    d. sun protector use

    D

17. What is **NOT** true of traditional day creams?
    a. the skin absorbs them poorly
    b. they tend to be mostly moisturizing
    c. they tend to be light
    d. they prepare the skin for makeup

    A

18. What are also referred to as nourishing creams?
    a. neck creams
    b. traditional night creams
    c. traditional day creams
    d. eye creams

    B

19. What should the client do before applying a night cream?
    a. heat the skin with a warm towel
    b. apply foundation makeup
    c. thoroughly cleanse the skin
    d. perform manual extractions

    C

20. What is true of the neck and the décolletage ?
    a. they do not require skin care
    b. they rarely show the effects of aging
    c. creams do not work on these areas
    d. they show age more than the face

    D

21. How often should neck creams be massaged into the skin?
    a. twice daily   c. once per week
    b. once per day   d. twice monthly

    A

22. How often should eye creams be used?
    a. once daily   c. once weekly
    b. twice daily   d. twice weekly

    B

23. What do eye creams incorporate in order to help supplement the lack of oil production in the eye area?
    a. extra antioxidants   c. extra emollients
    b. fewer antioxidants   d. fewer emollients

    C

24. What term refers to the form that eye creams are increasingly taking as the creams are designed to firm the eye area and reduce fine lines and wrinkles?
    a. nourishing creams   c. antioxidants
    b. astringents   d. treatment serums

    D

25. What is **NOT** among the conditions body creams are designed to relieve?
    a. severe dryness   c. "light arms"
    b. ingrown hair   d. "heavy legs"

    C

26. Where does one find the difference between creams and lotions?
    a. texture   c. color
    b. performance ingredients   d. skin care uses

    A

27. Why should you avoid applying lotions by placing the product on the palm of one hand, rubbing your hands together, and then patting the client's face with both hands?
    a. only one hand should be used so the other is free to wipe excess product
    b. more product stays on the palms of the hands than on the face
    c. product should be poured onto the skin directly from the container
    d. facial products have damaging effects on the skin of the palms

    B

28. What is another name for moisturizers?
    a. antioxidants   c. emulsifiers
    b. astringents   d. hydrators   D

29. What products are ideal mediums for incorporating a wide range
    of antioxidants as well as other appropriate botanicals for numerous
    benefits?
    a. moisturizers   c. lotions
    b. creams   d. ampoules   A

30. What term refers to products that contain concentrated ingredients,
    often in liposomes or other advanced delivery systems?
    a. lotions   c. creams
    b. serums   d. moisturizers   B

31. What is **NOT** among the specialty ingredients commonly found in
    serums?
    a. antioxidants   c. sunless tanners
    b. peptides   d. lipids   C

32. What is **NOT** true of masks?
    a. they are formulated with less water than creams, lotions,
       and fluids
    b. they can be peeled off
    c. they can be rinsed off
    d. they are lighter than creams, lotions, and fluids   D

33. What type of skin might be improved by a mask containing
    bentonine and kaolin?
    a. oily   c. sensitive
    b. normal   d. dry   A

34. What condition might be improved by a mask containing sulfur,
    salicylic acid, or benzoyl peroxide, plus botanicals for healing,
    soothing, and antiseptic action?
    a. hyperpigmentation   c. hypopigmentation
    b. acne   d. albinism   B

35. What type of skin might be improved by a mask containing large
    amounts of emollients?
    a. oily   c. dry
    b. sun-damaged   d. couperose   C

CHAPTER 15—PHARMACOLOGY FOR ESTHETICIANS

1. What is a serious hypersensitive allergic reaction characterized by respiratory distress, hypotension, edema, rash, and tachycardia?
   a. anaphylaxis
   b. angina
   c. anorexia
   d. acute coronary syndrome

   A

2. What is an antacid?
   a. any fungus that results in disease
   b. any agent that neutralizes stomach acid
   c. a fungal infection below the skin
   d. any pharmaceutical painkiller

   B

3. What term refers to a class of drugs used to prevent the onset of an anginal attack?
   a. antithrombotics   c. antianginals
   b. antiemetics   d. antiretrovirals

   C

4. What term refers to a class of drugs used to limit spasms and cramping, particularly of the digestive and urinary tracts?
   a. antianginals   c. antiemetics
   b. anticonvulsants   d. anticholinergics

   D

5. What term refers to a class of drugs used to prevent or limit the severity of spastic activity resulting from certain neurological conditions?
   a. anticonvulsants   c. antihistamines
   b. antiretrovirals   d. antiemetics

   A

6. What is a heart condition characterized by irregular heartbeats?
   a. acute coronary syndrome   c. anorexia
   b. arrhythmia   d. angina

   B

7. What term refers to a class of drugs with a sedative effect, predominantly used to treat anxiety and sleep disorders?
   a. inhibitors   c. benzodiazepines
   b. antithrombotics   d. tricyclics

   C

8. What term refers to an ocular condition characterized by fluid leaking from the macula, resulting in blurred vision?
   a. hypertrichosis   c. myocardial ischemia
   b. metabolic alkalosis   d. central serous retinopathy

   D

9. What term refers to a condition characterized by symptoms including low mood, loss of interest, loss of energy, weight changes, and possible thoughts of suicide?
   a. depression
   b. hallucination
   c. epilepsy
   d. hypertension

   A

10. Where in the body does a dowager's hump form because of slow bone loss over time?
    a. inside the rib cage
    b. along the spine
    c. under the jaw
    d. around the knee

    B

11. What does the term "efficacy" mean?
    a. ability of a drug to retain potency over a long time
    b. probability of side effects
    c. ability of a treatment or drug to produce a specific result
    d. probability of allergic reactions

    C

12. What is epilepsy?
    a. state of increased alkalines in the body resulting from decreased acids
    b. ocular condition marked by fluid leaking from the macula
    c. condition marked by unspecific or unwarranted anxiety
    d. neurological condition characterized by sudden seizures

    D

13. What is generalized anxiety disorder?
    a. condition characterized by unspecific or unwarranted anxiety
    b. neurological condition characterized by sudden seizures
    c. state of increased alkalines in the body resulting from decreased acids
    d. ocular condition marked by fluid leaking from the macula

    A

14. What are hallucinations?
    a. chest pains resulting from lack of oxygen to the heart
    b. abnormal visions associated with certain psychoses
    c. ocular conditions marked by fluid leaking from the macula
    d. sudden seizures resulting from a neurological condition

    B

15. What is a virus transmitted to humans through mice feces with potentially fatal consequences?
    a. mycosis
    b. angina
    c. hantavirus
    d. ischemia

    C

16. What is hypertrichosis?
    a. excessive hair growth where hair does not normally grow
    b. chest pain resulting from lack of oxygen to the heart
    c. a neurological condition marked by sudden seizures
    d. an ocular condition marked by fluid leaking from the macula

    A

17. What term refers to limited or reduced functioning of the immune system?
    a. autoimmune   c. pathogenic
    b. immunocompromised   d. parenteral

    B

18. What is a state of increased alkalines in the body resulting from decreased acids?
    a. alkalinity   c. metabolic alkalosis
    b. anaphylaxis   d. myocardial ischemia

    C

19. What term refers to a class of drugs used to treat depression?
    a. selective seratonin reuptake
    b. bronchodilators
    c. benzodiazepines inhibitors
    d. monoamine oxidase inhibitors

    D

20. What term refers to any infection or disease caused by a fungus that invades the tissues, causing superficial, subcutaneous, or systemic disease?
    a. mycosis   c. anorexia
    b. epilepsy   d. placebo

    A

21. What is a neurotransmitter responsible for heart rate and the fight-or-flight reaction?
    a. imodium   c. norepinephrine
    b. lidocaine   d. Retin-A

    C

22. What is an anxiety disorder characterized by perpetual and excessive thoughts and activities that interfere with the normal functioning of the affected individual?
    a. post-traumatic stress disorder
    b. phobia
    c. depression
    d. obsessive-compulsive disorder

    D

23. What is a characteristic of osteoarthritis?
    a. inflammation of weight-bearing joints
    b. hardening of the arteries
    c. loss of bone density
    d. weakening of muscle tissues

    A

24. What term refers to piercing of mucous membranes or the skin barrier through such events as needlesticks, human bites, and abrasions?
    a. subcutaneous   c. autoimmune
    b. parenteral   d. pathogenic

    B

25. What is a pathogenic fungus?
    a. any naturally occurring fungus
    b. a fungal infection below the skin
    c. any fungus that results in disease
    d. a fungus found only in the stomach

    C

26. What term refers to the wearing down of stomach and esophagus tissue, resulting in frequent stomach pain, especially after eating?
    a. peptic ulcer   c. hypertrichosis
    b. pathogenic fungi   d. hypertension

    A

27. What term refers to a persistent, irrational fear of a specific or particular object or situation or activity that compels a desire to avoid it?
    a. obsessive-compulsive disorder
    b. phobia
    c. post-traumatic stress disorder
    d. anxiety

    B

28. What is photosensitivity?
    a. aversion to being photographed
    b. another term for hyperpigmentation
    c. responsiveness to sunlight
    d. another term for hypopigmentation

    C

29. What term refers to a substance having no pharmacological effect, but administered as a control in testing the efficacy of a biologically active preparation?
    a. imodium   c. lamisil
    b. remova   d. placebo

    D

30. What is post-traumatic stress disorder?
    a. mental condition
    b. physical condition
    c. allergic reaction
    d. congenital defect

    A

31. What term refers to a type of antidepressant that allows for more productive use of a particular neurotransmitter?
    a. monoamine oxidase inhibitors
    b. selective seratonin reuptake inhibitors
    c. bronchodilators
    d. benzodiazepines

    B

32. What does the term "sublingual" mean?
    a. behind the ear
    b. above the eye
    c. under the tongue
    d. around the nipple

    C

33. What skin condition results from the introduction of vegetative matter to an open wound, leading to infection that is limited to the dermis?
    a. subcutaneous mycosis
    b. opportunistic mycosis
    c. systemic micosis
    d. superficial mycosis

    D

34. What is the most commonly prescribed type of antidepressant used to treat milder cases of depression or anxiety?
    a. tricyclics
    b. inhibitors
    c. benzodiazepines
    d. antithrombotics

    A

35. What term refers to a type of chemical dependence in which the affected individual thinks he or she needs a substance in order to function?
    a. chemical dependence
    b. psychological dependence
    c. physical dependence
    d. pharmaceutical dependence

    B

Part 4: Advanced Esthetics

CHAPTER 16—ADVANCED FACIAL TECHNIQUES

1. What is a treatment consideration for dehydrated skin?
   a. oily skin has become impacted
   b. the stratum corneum is resistive to the penetration of products
   c. the client cannot be expected to perform complex home care
   d. products that will further inflame the skin must be avoided   _B_

2. What is **NOT** one of the elements of a client history?
   a. education level   c. allergies
   b. medical conditions   d. contraindications   _A_

3. What additional process continues during the basic cleansing step of a treatment?
   a. extractions   c. application of masks
   b. skin analysis   d. application of sunscreen   _B_

4. What type of product will vary depending on whether your goal is to strip, pH balance, hydrate, or soothe the skin?
   a. cleanser   c. toner
   b. sunscreen   d. moisturizer   _C_

5. What treatment step can be administered with compresses, a spray device, a steamer, or wet towels?
   a. basic cleanse   c. water/moisture
   b. mask   d. protection   _D_

6. What is a treatment consideration for clogged skin?
   a. the client cannot be expected to perform complex home care
   b. products that will further inflame the skin must be avoided
   c. oily skin has become impacted
   d. the stratum corneum is resistive to the penetration of products   _C_

7. What treatment step involves the use of acids, enzymes, equipment, and/or scrubs?
   a. exfoliation   c. basic cleanse
   b. water/moisture   d. protection   _A_

8. What treatment step may be skipped altogether for acne-prone or severely damaged skin?
   a. basic cleanse   c. toner
   b. massage   d. water/moisture   _B_

9. What is **NOT** one of the penetration techniques for specialty serums?
   a. ultrasound
   b. alginate masks
   c. hypodermic injection
   d. microcurrent

   C

10. What is a treatment consideration for young teenage skin?
    a. the stratum corneum is resistive to the penetration of products
    b. oily skin has become impacted
    c. products that will further inflame the skin must be avoided
    d. the client cannot be expected to perform complex home care

    D

11. What treatment step helps seal in your great work?
    a. penetration of ampoules
    b. massage
    c. toner
    d. protection

    D

12. What type of skin would benefit from massage that is followed by ultrasound, iontophoresis, or microcurrent?
    a. dehydrated skin
    b. teenage skin
    c. clogged skin
    d. oily skin

    A

13. What is a treatment consideration for sensitive skin?
    a. products that will further inflame the skin must be avoided
    b. the stratum corneum is resistive to the penetration of products
    c. negative galvanic current may be applied
    d. skin impactions and may require softening

    A

14. What is good SPF measurement for sunscreen applied to dehydrated skin?
    a. at least 7
    b. at least 15
    c. at least 21
    d. at least 30

    B

15. What is the key to treating clogged skin?
    a. introducing moisture with both steam and hydrating serums
    b. performing harsh exfoliation
    c. softening the impactions for extraction
    d. avoiding inflaming the skin

    C

16. When should toner be applied to clogged skin?
    a. before extraction
    b. before cleanser
    c. before protection
    d. after extraction

    D

17. What tools should be used for performing gentle extractions on clogged skin?
    a. cotton swabs
    b. lancets
    c. exfoliating scrubs
    d. tongs

    A

18. What product can be pushed deeper into clogged skin with negative galvanic current?
    a. non-oily hydration fluid
    b. desincrustant lotion
    c. soothing serum
    d. clay-based cleansing mask

    B

19. What is a good strategy for advising young teenage clients about proper home care?
    a. cover everything possible
    b. avoid specifics
    c. keep it simple
    d. young clients do not need home care

    C

20. What is the best way to help young clients prevent future sun damage?
    a. recommend staying out of the sun
    b. suggest wearing hats regularly
    c. suggest growing very long hair
    d. encourage the daily use of sunscreen

    D

21. How frequently do most prepubescent teens require treatment until further development of the pore structure or the beginning of acne flare-ups?
    a. bimonthly   c. weekly
    b. biweekly   d. daily

    A

22. How often should salon treatments be scheduled for older teenagers, except in cases of more severe acne?
    a. weekly   c. bimonthly
    b. monthly   d. annually

    B

23. What can be used to presoften the clogged areas of a teenager's skin?
    a. chemical exfoliant   c. desincrustant solution
    b. gentle cleanser   d. mild toner

    C

24. What is generally **NOT** appropriate for use on sensitive skin?
    a. soothing serum   c. iontophoresis
    b. cool cryoglobes   d. exfoliation

    D

25. What ensures that a client does not leave the clinic with a pink or red face?
    a. finishing mask   c. iontophoresis
    b. basic cleanse   d. non-oily hydration fluid

    A

26. What should you do before removing a hardened clay-based mask, in order to avoid irritating the client's skin?
    a. heat the mask with a blowdryer
    b. prewet the mask
    c. crack the mask with a metal spoon
    d. rub the mask with ice

    B

27. What do warm, wet towels add to treatment that helps improve product penetration?
    a. exfoliation   c. occlusion
    b. extraction   d. protection

    C

28. What condition is a contraindication for the use of warm towels?
    a. vitiligo   c. hypopigmentation
    b. hyperpigmentation   d. rosacea

    D

29. What statement about allergies is true?
    a. any given ingredient can cause an allergic reaction
    b. ingredients for sensitive skin do not cause allergic reactions
    c. all clients are allergic to a variety of ingredients
    d. only chemical ingredients cause allergic reactions

    A

30. What are the number one cause of cosmetic skin allergies?
    a. cleansers   c. latex gloves
    b. fragrances   d. toners

    B

31. What can be used to soothe the skin after an allergic reaction?
    a. low-pH exfoliation chemicals   c. atomized water
    b. carbonated water   d. alcohol-based products

    C

32. What is **NOT** an appropriate treatment adjustment for a client using retinoids?
    a. using fragrance-free hydrators
    b. avoiding stimulating products
    c. discontinuing exfoliation
    d. adding alcohol-based products

    D

33. What is **NOT** an example of a clinic exfoliation treatment?
    a. the use of a spray device
    b. equipment exfoliation
    c. manual microdermabrasion
    d. the use of enzymes

    A

34. What technique is rather like a classic scrub on steroids?
    a. iontophoresis
    b. manual microdermabrasion
    c. cool cryoglobes
    d. microcurrent

    B

35. What does the term "proteolytic" mean?
    a. comedogenic
    b. noncomedogenic
    c. protein-dissolving
    d. protein-stimulating

    C

CHAPTER 17—ADVANCED SKIN CARE MASSAGE

1. What term refers to the practice of inserting fine needles through the skin to specific points in order to help relieve pain or cure disease?
    a. acupuncture
    c. reflexology
    b. acupressure
    d. shiatsu

    A

2. Where did acupuncture originate?
    a. Japan
    c. Korea
    b. China
    d. Thailand

    B

3. What term refers to a common gray-to-black fine-grained volcanic rock?
    a. mastoid
    c. basalt
    b. sedimentary
    d. quartz

    C

4. What term refers to the belief that the health of the entire organism is reflected in each individual part of the organism?
    a. reflexology
    c. mastoid process
    b. conduction
    d. microorganism

    A

5. What should massage be viewed as?
    a. healing practice
    c. chemical treatment
    b. surgical procedure
    d. herbal therapy

    A

6. What should you do if you doubt whether a client is suitable for massage?
    a. ask the client to make the decision about performing massage
    b. get clearance from the client's physician
    c. perform massage, but use only very gentle techniques
    d. perform the normal massage routine

    B

7. How much time should pass after a client receives a facial injection before the client can safely receive facial massage?
    a. two hours
    c. two weeks
    b. two days
    d. two months

    C

8. What is **NOT** one of the terms that refer to blood clots?
    a. thrombolysis
    c. mastoid
    b. thrombosis
    d. embolus

    D

9. What commonly occurs when a client with high blood pressure becomes overheated?
    a. headache
    c. acne breakout
    b. nausea
    d. allergic reaction

    A

10. What is true about clients with cancer?
    a. they cannot receive massage
    b. they benefit from massage
    c. massage is contraindicated only during chemotherapy
    d. massage is contraindicated only during radiation treatments

    B

11. What is **NOT** one of the key components of a good massage?
    a. fluidity
    b. continuity
    c. reflexology
    d. suitability

    C

12. What is the **BEST** reason for varying your massage technique slightly from time to time?
    a. to prevent edema
    b. to ensure that you use various products before they expire
    c. to justify price increases
    d. so clients do not find your work predictable

    D

13. What should you do if a client comments that he or she especially enjoys a specific massage movement?
    a. include the specific movement every time you treat that client
    b. eliminate all other movements from the client's treatment
    c. charge extra to perform that specific movement in the future
    d. assume that all clients will react in the exact same way

    A

14. What is a primary concern when adding a new movement into your existing procedure?
    a. stopping the treatment to explain the new movement
    b. ensuring that the movement fits into the flow of the massage
    c. trying the movement on several parts of the client's body
    d. ensuring that you never give the same massage twice

    B

15. What does the term "shiatsu" mean?
    a. digital pressure
    b. digital manipulation
    c. finger pressure
    d. finger manipulation

    C

16. What is the Chinese word for the energy circulating throughout the body?
    a. *ko*
    b. *ki*
    c. *qo*
    d. *qi*

    D

17. What are the energy pathways in the body called, according to traditional Chinese medicine?
    a. meridians
    b. mastoids
    c. nasolabial grooves
    d. infraorbital ridges

    A

18. What is combined with massage techniques during Shiatsu treatments?
    a. therapeutic use of needles
    b. pressure on energy points
    c. essential-oil aromatherapy
    d. aggressive exfoliation

    B

19. What is true of Shiatsu massage?
    a. it requires special equipment
    b. it requires special oils
    c. it can be performed on a daily basis
    d. it is very difficult to learn

    C

20. What is the first step for each touch in Shiatsu?
    a. insert needle   c. release pressure
    b. apply pressure   d. touch the skin

    D

21. What is the last step for each touch in Shiatsu massage?
    a. release pressure   c. insert needle
    b. apply pressure   d. touch the skin

    A

22. What technique is **NOT** based on the microsystems theory?
    a. foot reflexology   c. pulse diagnosis
    b. lymph drainage   d. iridology

    B

23. What are stones used for in the esthetic arena?
    a. their ability to cure disease
    b. their ability to repair skin damage
    c. their ability to relax clients
    d. their ability to enhance beauty

    C

24. What triggers vasoconstriction, which blanches the skin and reduces inflammation?
    a. paraffin wax treatments
    b. thermal mask treatments
    c. placing warm stones on the skin
    d. placing cold stones on the skin

    D

25. What can reduce redness after waxing?
    a. applying cold stones   c. vigorous massage
    b. applying warm stones   d. gentle massage

    A

26. What should you do after removing stones from a heater?
    a. immediately apply them to the client's skin
    b. let them cool on a towel until you can hold them comfortably
    c. hand them to the client so the client can appraise the temperature
    d. place them in a refrigerator for a quick cool down

    B

27. What should you do after you have completed using a stone during a treatment?
    a. discard the stone because it is soiled
    b. toss the stone into a nearby sink
    c. place the stone on a towel
    d. put the stone into your pocket

    C

28. Where should stones be positioned in relation to the client's spine?
    a. just above the spine
    b. just below the spine
    c. directly on the spine
    d. on either side of the spine

    D

29. Why are larger stones impractical for facial manipulations?
    a. they do not fit the facial contours well
    b. they cause bruising
    c. they retain excessive amounts of cold and/or heat
    d. they cause excessive discomfort on the face

    A

30. When using the technique that involves a hot stone in one hand and a cold stone in the other, what is the order in which the stones are applied?
    a. cold stone leads, hot stone follows
    b. hot stone leads, cold stone follows
    c. both are applied simultaneously
    d. hot and cold should not be mixed

    B

31. What can be very distracting to the client?
    a. gently opening and closing the door to the stone heater
    b. softly asking a client if stone temperature is acceptable
    c. placing a used stone onto a towel for storage
    d. clanking or dropping stones during treatment

    D

32. When did Dr. Emil Vodder originally develop modern lymphatic drainage techniques?
    a. late 1830s   c. late 1930s
    b. early 1890s   d. early 1980s

    C

33. What effectively reduces bruising and edema following injury or surgery, including dental and cosmetic surgery?
    a. lymphatic drainage massage
    b. cold stone therapy
    c. warm stone therapy
    d. vigorous massage

    A

34. What is **NOT** one of the causes of facial edema?
    a. weeping
    b. laughing
    c. infection
    d. injury

    B

35. How does lymphatic drainage massage benefit clients with low energy?
    a. by increasing hemoglobin production
    b. by toning the muscles
    c. by stimulating immune circulation
    d. by triggering adrenaline release

    C

CHAPTER 18—ADVANCED FACIAL DEVICES

1. What term refers to pink, sometimes scaly, abnormal skin lesions that are considered precancerous?
    a. actinic keratosis
    b. cellulitis
    c. impetigo
    d. vitiligo

    A

2. What term describes the state of ultramicroscopic particles suspended in the air of a gas?
    a. compressed
    b. aerosolized
    c. condensed
    d. ablative

    B

3. What term refers to a psychological disease that causes individuals to be inappropriately concerned, obsessed, or fixated with their appearance?
    a. electrodesiccation
    b. dyschromia
    c. body dysmorphic disorder
    d. selective photothermolysis

    C

4. What term refers to a potentially serious infection of the skin that presents as a small, red area surrounding a skin injury?
    a. impetigo
    b. vitiligo
    c. actinic keratosis
    d. cellulitis

    D

5. What term refers to an abnormal display of facial hyperpigmentation due to solar damage?
    a. dyschromia
    b. electrodesiccation
    c. body dysmorphic disorder
    d. selective photothermolysis

    A

6. What is a therapy that uses a device that emits low levels of radiofrequency and high-frequency current in order to dry or destroy a targeted superficial lesion?
    a. selective photothermolysis
    b. electrodesiccation
    c. dyschromia
    d. intense pulsed light

    B

7. What term refers to a topical medication that is used for bleaching or reducing excessive melanin lesions in the epidermis?
    a. poikiloderma
    b. nikolski
    c. hydroquinone
    d. dyschromia

    C

8. What term refers to a contagious skin infection caused by stapphylococcal or strepococcal bacteria?
   a. vitiligo
   b. actinic keratosis
   c. cellulitis
   d. impetigo

   _D_

9. One microampere is equivalent to _____ of an ampere.
   a. one-millionth
   b. one-thousandth
   c. one-hundredth
   d. one-tenth

   _A_

10. What is a Nikolski sign?
    a. a warning label on a device
    b. an indication of a skin reaction
    c. a hand signal from a client
    d. a poster in the treatment room

    _B_

11. What term describes a procedure in which the epidermis remains intact and no resulting skin vaporization or trauma occurs?
    a. noncomedogenic
    b. comedogenic
    c. nonablative
    d. ablative

    _C_

12. What term refers to the mottled redness or brown discoloration appearing most commonly in women on the sides of the neck or the upper chest?
    a. sebaceous hyperplasia
    b. pseudofolliculitis barbae
    c. Nevus of Ota
    d. Poikiloderma of Civatte

    _D_

13. What is another term for pulse duration?
    a. pulse width
    b. pulse length
    c. pulse term
    d. pulse scope

    _A_

14. What term refers to treatment using an appropriate wavelength, exposure time, and pulse duration, with sufficient energy fluence to absorb light into a specific area?
    a. electrodesiccation
    b. selective photothermolysis
    c. dyschromia
    d. photorejuvenation

    _B_

15. What is splattering?
    a. singed skin
    b. discolored skin
    c. singed hair
    d. discolored hair

    _C_

16. What term is used to measure heat contained in a chromophore?
    a. ampere
    b. microampere
    c. thermal coefficient
    d. thermal storage

    _D_

17. What is **NOT** one of the key factors upon which purchasing decisions about products and treatments need to be based?
    a. advertisement claims
    b. legalities
    c. business goals
    d. financial opportunities

    _A_

18. What information should you acquire from your state licensing board and/or regulatory agencies when researching an equipment purchase?
    a. which products will give you the best long-term value
    b. whether particular procedures are within your scope of practice
    c. how much you should budget each year for equipment purchase
    d. whether a particular procedure will remain popular with clients

    _B_

19. What may you need to do if your market cannot bear the price that you will need to charge to pay for a particular service?
    a. raise all of your other prices
    b. eliminate less expensive services
    c. reconsider the purchase of the equipment used to offer the service
    d. relocate your business

    _C_

20. Why is it important to review the predominant skin type and demographic information of your clientele before purchasing a new device?
    a. this step is unnecessary because all devices work for all clients
    b. very few clients have skin that is appropriate for device treatment
    c. to negotiate a better purchase price
    d. some laser/light devices are safe only for specific skin types

    _D_

21. What is **NOT** one of the factors to consider when making a purchase decision for an esthetics device?
    a. packaging
    b. specifications
    c. configuration
    d. upgrade capabilities

    _A_

22. What type of equipment is eligible for marketing tools and system upgrades?
    a. used equipment
    b. new equipment
    c. both new and used equipment
    d. neither new nor used equipment

    _B_

23. Why should you negotiate a reputable maintenance and service contract when purchasing a used device?
    a. every used device is guaranteed to break within a year of purchase
    b. most sellers of used equipment are dishonest about item quality
    c. the original warranty is usually invalidated by third-party sale
    d. purchasing this sort of contract is actually an unnecessary expense

    _C_

24. What term refers to a contractual stipulation that allows you to prematurely terminate a lease?
    a. exit strategy
    b. back door
    c. termination agreement
    d. escape clause

    _D_

25. What document can help determine whether the operation of the device falls within the esthetician's scope of practice?
    a. intended use statement
    b. warranty
    c. instruction manual
    d. assembly directions

    _A_

26. Why is education from a company sales representative sometimes inappropriate?
    a. most representatives will be dishonest in order to make a sale
    b. representatives who are not skin care specialists lack information
    c. representatives only offer training at their corporate headquarters
    d. representatives charge large fees for providing training

    _B_

27. What is the standard term for the warranty that comes with a laser, IPL, or RF device?
    a. 30 days
    b. six months
    c. one year
    d. five years

    _C_

28. How many preventative maintenance (PM) checks per year are recommended for laser, IPL, or RF devices?
    a. eight
    b. six
    c. four
    d. two

    _D_

29. What is **NOT** among the common conditions that can be treated with an IPL device and photorejuvenation?
    a. adult onset acne
    b. small spider veins
    c. pigmented lesions
    d. fine lines and wrinkles

    _A_

30. Who should supervise the operation of IPL devices?
    a. state licensing inspector
    b. physician
    c. manufacturer's representative
    d. esthetics educator

    B

31. What is the first step in the consultation for a potential facial-rejuvenation client?
    a. evaluate the client's skin type
    b. determine the client's goals
    c. take a thorough medical history
    d. ask about medications

    C

32. What is the last step in the consultation for a potential facial-rejuvenation client?
    a. take a thorough medical history
    b. ask about medications
    c. determine the client's goals
    d. ask about tanning history

    D

33. What is **NOT** a "red flag" that may come up during the consultation process with a client seeking photorejuvenation?
    a. a client with reasonable expectations of treatment results
    b. a client who gains all of his or her knowledge from the Internet
    c. a client who chronically moves from clinic to clinic
    d. a client who seems inappropriately fixated on his or her appearance

    A

34. What is **NOT** among the contraindications for photorejuvenation?
    a. photosensitivity to sunlight
    b. Accutane use over two years ago
    c. history of keloid formation
    d. suspicious skin lesions

    B

35. What color hair is a normal mode Nd-YAG laser effective for removing?
    a. light red   c. dark
    b. blonde   d. light brown

    C

CHAPTER 19—ADVANCED HAIR REMOVAL

1. What is the process by which heat causes cells to congeal and become dysfunctional?
    a. electrocoagulation
    b. ionization
    c. electrolysis
    d. hypertrichosis
    ____

2. What is the Egyptian word for threading?
    a. khite
    b. fatlah
    c. shiatsu
    d. ayurveda
    ____

3. What type of current is used in galvanic electrolysis?
    a. high-intensity current
    b. microcurrent
    c. direct current
    d. alternating current
    ____

4. What is the proper term for the process of physically changing to the opposite gender?
    a. transgenderism
    b. transvestitism
    c. hirsutism
    d. gender reassignment
    ____

5. What is a cutaneous viral infection commonly caused by sexual transmission and exhibited by genital warts?
    a. human papillomavirus
    b. hypertrichosis
    c. thermolysis
    d. diathermy
    ____

6. What term refers to the outer folds of the vulva on either side of the vagina?
    a. labia minora
    b. labia majora
    c. pedicle
    d. perineum
    ____

7. What term refers to the inner folds of the vulva on the edge of the vaginal opening?
    a. perineum
    b. labia majora
    c. labia minora
    d. pedicle
    ____

8. What part of the body is operated on during a rhinoplasty?
    a. stomach
    b. breasts
    c. chin
    d. nose
    ____

9. What term refers to genital surgery in which the testicles are removed and the skin from the penis is inverted to form a female sex organ?
    a. vaginoplasty
    b. rhinoplasty
    c. thermolysis
    d. diathermy
    ____

10. What is a method that uses alternating current to produce oscillating high-frequency radio waves?
   a. hypertrichosis
   b. thermolysis
   c. electrocoagulation
   d. ionization

11. What is another term for thermolysis?
   a. ionization
   b. electrocoagulation
   c. diathermy
   d. rhinoplasty

12. What helps you answer clients' questions and advise them about more advanced methods such as laser hair reduction and electrolysis?
   a. relying solely on what you learned while you were an esthetics student
   b. reading beauty magazines for tips about new fashion trends
   c. learning terminology that makes you sound informed
   d. understanding all current methods of hair removal

13. What is an effective method of increasing your potential for profit?
   a. learning and offering a broad range of services
   b. offering only the most expensive possible services
   c. rushing through treatments to handle extra clients
   d. raising prices without updating your service menu

14. What must you learn about in order to avoid malpractice liability?
   a. benefits associated with services
   b. risks associated with services
   c. how to represent yourself in court
   d. how to cut corners without the client noticing

15. What is true about happy, regular, repeat clients?
   a. they take up too much time
   b. they expect steep discounts
   c. they often provide referrals
   d. they eventually stop tipping

16. What is true of any circumstance in which hair is extracted from skin?
   a. blood is always released, but not lymph
   b. lymph is always released, but not blood
   c. body fluids are never released
   d. there is potential for body fluid release

17. What disorder presents as an ulceration on the genitals?
   a. herpes simplex virus
   b. hypertrichosis
   c. hirsutism
   d. hypopigmentation

18. What is the most common sexually transmitted disease?
    a. syphilis   c. AIDS
    b. genital herpes   d. gonorrhea   _____

19. Why is transmission of human papillomavirus (HPV) easy?
    a. it is an airborne virus
    b. it is a waterborne virus
    c. it is present in the food supply
    d. infection can go unnoticed   _____

20. How many types of HPV have scientists identified?
    a. fewer than 50   c. more than 100
    b. approximately 75   d. more than 200   _____

21. Why is hemophilia a contraindication for waxing treatments?
    a. bleeding can occur
    b. treatments aggravate sensitivity
    c. bruising can occur
    d. hemophiliacs feel pain easily   _____

22. What is **NOT** a contraindication for waxing?
    a. diabetes   c. epilepsy
    b. asthma   d. lupus   _____

23. When is it acceptable to wax eyelids, inside the ears or nose, or the
    areola of the breast?
    a. with physician's permission   c. always
    b. with client's permission   d. never   _____

24. What is true of a woman with a small amount of blond vellus hair on
    the upper lip or chin that is visible only in an 8-diopter mirror?
    a. she has hypertrichosis
    b. she has hirsutism
    c. her hair growth is normal
    d. her hair growth is abnormal   _____

25. What can cause hypertrichosis?
    a. pregnancy
    b. androgen dependence
    c. minor injury
    d. diseases of the endocrine system   _____

26. What can cause hirsutism?
    a. puberty
    b. genetic inheritance
    c. cancer treatments
    d. certain prescription medications   ____

27. What is another term for threading?
    a. coiling   c. banding
    b. gathering   d. stringing   ____

28. Where did the practice of threading originate?
    a. North America   c. Pacific Islands
    b. South America   d. Middle East   ____

29. Why is the plucking sensation of threading more tolerable for most
    clients than the plucking sensation of tweezing?
    a. hairs are snagged faster
    b. the removal angle is more direct
    c. many hairs are snagged at once
    d. the hair is snagged closer to the skin   ____

30. Why should you avoid creams when preparing a client's face for
    threading?
    a. creams will seep into pores and cause infections
    b. creams can reduce the gripping effectiveness of the thread
    c. creams harden the hairs and cause them to break during
       threading
    d. creams react to the friction of threading and heat the skin   ____

31. What should you use to perform threading?
    a. thick copper wire
    b. soft strand of yarn
    c. cotton household thread
    d. length of dental floss   ____

32. What is a good thread length for a threading procedure?
    a. 2 to 3 inches   c. 15 to 20 inches
    b. 6 to 12 inches   d. 24 to 30 inches   ____

33. What is **NOT** a contraindication for threading?
    a. oily skin   c. active psoriasis
    b. broken skin   d. sunburned skin   ____

34. What ancient people believed that body hair was unacceptable and unclean?
    a. Chinese   c. Hebrews
    b. Egyptians   d. Japanese   ____

35. What is true of hair regrown after sugaring?
    a. it is more coarse than before
    b. it is more dense than before
    c. it is lighter than before
    d. hair does not regrow after sugaring   ____

CHAPTER 20—ADVANCED MAKEUP

1. What does the world of makeup offer clients that they cannot receive from skin care?
   a. immediate results
   b. treatment for conditions
   c. thorough cleansing
   d. exfoliation ____

2. What has titanium dioxide been approved for by the FDA?
   a. exfoliation
   b. cleansing
   c. sun protection
   d. toning ____

3. What is true of makeup-related services in the salon?
   a. they take time away from more profitable services
   b. they can be one of your highest profit centers
   c. they do not generate many sales
   d. most clients avoid mixing makeup and skin treatments ____

4. Who generally has a happy experience during a makeup service?
   a. only the client
   b. only the makeup artist
   c. both the client and the makeup artist
   d. neither the client nor the makeup artist ____

5. What is the primary ingredient of most non-mineral color cosmetics?
   a. boron nitride
   b. bismuth oxychloride
   c. alcohol
   d. talcum powder ____

6. What word, used to describe minerals in powders, means that something cannot support bacterial life?
   a. inert
   b. ablative
   c. comedogenic
   d. alkaline ____

7. What is **NOT** a known sensitizer?
   a. FD&C dye
   b. mineral powder
   c. synthetic fragrance
   d. synthetic preservative ____

8. What has zinc oxide been approved for by the FDA?
   a. antibacterial agent
   b. exfoliating agent
   c. chemical sunscreen
   d. physical sunscreen ____

9. What is called "synthetic pearl" because of its metallic sheen?
   a. bismuth oxychloride
   b. boron nitride
   c. titanium dioxide
   d. zinc oxide ____

10. What is true of minerals in mineral powders?
   a. they are granulated soil
   b. they are scientifically manipulated and/or entirely synthesized
   c. they are crushed pieces of rock
   d. they are scientifically processed botanical products ____

11. Why do mineral powders provide excellent coverage with very little product?
   a. they cling to the skin better than talc-based makeup
   b. powder grains expand on contact with human skin
   c. they are concentrated pigment
   d. they change the client's skin type ____

12. What is **NOT** one of the ways minerals interact with light?
   a. minerals reflect light   c. minerals diffuse light
   b. minerals refract light   d. minerals block light ____

13. Why is it important to try minerals on the skin to test for color rather than make a decision based on the color in the jar?
   a. minerals interact with light and blend with the skin
   b. minerals lose most of their color when removed from the jar
   c. minerals completely change color when they touch human skin
   d. jars are tinted to give a false impression of the product's color ____

14. What is true about the sun protection factor (SPF) of mineral makeup?
   a. all mineral makeup provides SPF
   b. only products that list SPF on the label provide sun protection
   c. no mineral makeup provides SPF
   d. products that list SPF on the label block all of the sun's radiation ____

15. How should properly applied mineral makeup feel on the skin?
   a. thick   c. weightless
   b. wet   d. sticky ____

16. What does the look of properly applied mineral makeup mimic the appearance of?
   a. sheer plastic   c. mature, healthy skin
   b. smooth silk   d. young, healthy skin ____

17. Where on the client's face should you perform a color test before application?
   a. jawline   c. right cheek
   b. left cheek   d. forehead ____

18. Why should you avoid using a brush with a large dome head when applying loose mineral powder?
    a. it will hurt the client's face
    b. it will scatter the powder
    c. it will absorb too much product
    d. it will not absorb enough product   ____

19. How should you treat the face when applying mineral powder with a brush?
    a. thirds   c. quadrants
    b. halves   d. eighths   ____

20. What effect can you achieve by using a lighter base in the aesthetic triangle and a darker one in the perimeter?
    a. downplaying a large nose
    b. downplaying a high forehead
    c. accentuating sensual lips
    d. "pulling out" the center of the face   ____

21. What tool should you use to blend minerals?
    a. flocked sponge   c. side of your hand
    b. damp paper towel   d. basic cosmetic sponge   ____

22. What is a reasonable goal when applying minerals for camouflage?
    a. making the facial distraction completely invisible
    b. normalizing the client's appearance as much as possible
    c. aiding the medical treatment process for the client's condition
    d. permanently improving the client's appearance   ____

23. What do some professional makeup artists use as a palette?
    a. side of a makeup box
    b. clean white towel
    c. back of a gloved hand
    d. smooth, pale-colored stone   ____

24. What type of light is best for finding the color that will cover redness on a client's skin?
    a. fluorescent light   c. LED light
    b. tungsten light   d. natural daylight   ____

25. What rule is true about applying mineral concealer to undereye circles?
    a. the darker the circle, the darker the concealer should be
    b. the darker the circle, the lighter the concealer should be
    c. foundation should be applied after the concealer
    d. yellow is the only color that works in this circumstance   ____

26. What is the weakest finger you have and therefore a good tool for blending concealer?
    a. thumb   c. middle finger
    b. ring finger   d. pinky   ____

27. How can you minimize a puff under the eye?
    a. apply a uniform color to the entire perimeter of the eye
    b. use a light color on the top eyelid
    c. graduate the color from light at the edges to darker in the middle
    d. use a dark color on the top eyelid   ____

28. What statement about scar tissue is correct?
    a. it is highly resistant to UV rays
    b. it contains numerous sweat glands
    c. it has a dark, dull appearance
    d. it contains no hair follicles   ____

29. What are your biggest challenges in camouflage?
    a. bruising and tattoos
    b. scars
    c. hyperpigmentation and vitiligo
    d. undereye discolorations   ____

30. What is **NOT** an ingredient of the most beneficial water-based liquid airbrush foundations?
    a. humectants   c. oil absorbers
    b. alcohol   d. vitamins   ____

31. What is true about alcohol-based liquid airbrush foundations?
    a. the alcohol evaporates slowly
    b. the final surface smudges easily
    c. the final surface is waterproof
    d. they offer a broad range of coverage   ____

32. What method of airbrush makeup application involves spraying the skin briefly with just air to indicate where the makeup will be applied?
    a. narrow spray pattern
    b. wide spray pattern
    c. dash method
    d. point-and-shoot/dot method   _____

33. How far from the skin is the narrow spray pattern applied?
    a. 1/4-inch to 3 inches   c. 4 to 7 inches
    b. 2 to 5 inches   d. 6 to 9 inches   _____

34. How far from the skin is the wide spray pattern applied?
    a. 1/4-inch to 3 inches   c. 6 to 9 inches
    b. 3 to 6 inches   d. more than 9 inches   _____

35. What term refers to the bubbling of liquid and air into the holding bowl of the airbrush during the mixing and cleaning process?
    a. back reservoir   c. back bubble
    b. holding reservoir   d. holding bubble   _____

Part 5: Spa and Alternative Therapies

CHAPTER 21—SPA TREATMENTS

1. What type of spa might offer body treatments, exercise classes, fitness facilities, medical treatments, and outdoor activities with client experiences lasting several days?
    a. destination spa
    b. day spa
    c. wellness center
    d. rehabilitation center
    ____

2. What type of spa might offer yoga, personal development seminars, Pilates, and weight-loss clinics?
    a. rehabilitation center
    b. wellness center
    c. destination spa
    d. day spa
    ____

3. What is a benefit of spa treatments?
    a. treating serious medical conditions
    b. treating psychiatric conditions
    c. revitalizing the spirit temporarily
    d. providing lasting improvement
    ____

4. When is it appropriate to leave a client unattended while a treatment is processing?
    a. during wrap treatments
    b. during hydrotherapy treatments
    c. when working with two clients simultaneously
    d. never
    ____

5. What is **NOT** an example of proper client confidentiality?
    a. discussing client information in public
    b. safeguarding personal information
    c. keeping information in a safe place
    d. sharing information with essential staff
    ____

6. How do you promote an open and comfortable place in which your clients will feel safe and protected?
    a. by openly discussing client conditions in the spa lobby
    b. by respecting clients' privacy and creating a trusting environment
    c. by inviting potential customers to observe ongoing treatments
    d. by sharing information about your last client with your current client
    ____

7. What is the **FIRST** step of the proper daily shutdown process?
   a. wipe down treatment tables
   b. replenish supplies
   c. put on gloves
   d. vacuum, mop, and spray the room _____

8. What function does the liquid soap base of an herbal scrub serve?
   a. soothing
   b. moisturizing
   c. skin cell regeneration
   d. cleansing _____

9. What happens when you apply products to large areas or the entire body, as opposed to simply applying products to the face?
   a. the safety concerns are exactly the same in both circumstances
   b. the risk of allergic reaction decreases
   c. the risk of allergic reaction or complication increases
   d. the risk of complications decreases _____

10. What is **NOT** among the possible contraindications for body treatments?
    a. open wounds
    b. sunburned skin
    c. claustrophobia
    d. asthma _____

11. Whose comfort should be taken into consideration when selecting a treatment table?
    a. the client's and the esthetician's
    b. only the client's
    c. only the esthetician's
    d. neither the client's nor the esthetician's _____

12. What purpose do cutouts in treatment tables serve?
    a. allowing the technician to reach underneath the client's body
    b. allowing the client to lie face down, as opposed to with the head turned
    c. letting the client extend his or her arms to the floor during treatment
    d. creating a comfortable space for the breasts of female clients _____

13. How many heads does a Vichy shower have?
    a. two
    b. three to five
    c. five to seven
    d. nine _____

14. When should estheticians wear gloves during spa treatments?
    a. only during extractions
    b. only during facial treatments
    c. only when working near the genitals
    d. always ____

15. What is **NOT** an example of a harmful bacteria that some individuals carry on the surface of their skin?
    a. HIV   c. salmonella
    b. CA-MRSA   d. *E. coli* ____

16. What term refers to a body treatment involving the application of an exfoliating, hydrating, detoxifying coating to the entire body?
    a. spa wrap   c. body wrap
    b. body mask   d. spa mask ____

17. What requires disinfection?
    a. any object in the salon
    b. any object that has been touched
    c. any object prepared for use
    d. any single-use object ____

18. What function does finely ground oat powder serve in an herbal scrub?
    a. soothing   c. cleansing
    b. skin cell regeneration   d. moisturizing ____

19. What is the **LAST** step of the daily shutdown process?
    a. put on gloves
    b. wipe down treatment tables
    c. replenish supplies
    d. vacuum, mop, and spray the room ____

20. What is the first step in preparing the client for a procedure?
    a. review the client's health history
    b. tell the client to remove jewelry
    c. tell the client to disrobe
    d. drape the client for modesty ____

21. Why should you have plenty of drinking water on hand in the treatment room?
    a. in case you get thirsty
    b. to protect clients from dehydration
    c. to help cool skin in emergencies
    d. to help clean off instruments ____

22. How many modesty towels should you provide for a female client who elects **NOT** to wear disposable undergarments during a treatment?
    a. six
    b. four
    c. two
    d. one ____

23. How should you adjust the towel when it is time for the client to roll from a prone or supine position?
    a. roll the towel down a tube below to the client's feet
    b. yank the towel off and hold it drooping from one hand
    c. the client should adjust the towel himself or herself
    d. lift the towel horizontally and extend your arms over your head ____

24. What term refers to a body treatment that integrates linens or elastic bandages infused with ingredients to reduce the appearance of cellulite or to hydrate the skin?
    a. body wrap
    b. body mask
    c. spa wrap
    d. spa mask ____

25. How can you ensure full absorption during an elastic wrap?
    a. soak the wrap after application
    b. heat the wrap after application
    c. soak the wrap in advance
    d. heat the wrap in advance ____

26. How long should a seaweed wrap process on the client's body?
    a. 10 minutes
    b. 15 minutes
    c. 30 minutes
    d. 45 minutes ____

27. What should a client do for 24 hours before and after a seaweed wrap?
    a. drink extra water
    b. stay awake
    c. eat extra amounts of salty foods
    d. refrain from eating ____

28. What function does honey serve in an herbal scrub?
    a. cleansing
    b. moisturizing
    c. soothing
    d. skin cell regeneration ____

29. What term refers to a unit designed to hold water and to heat linen wraps to an optimal temperature?
    a. Vichy shower
    b. moist-heat unit
    c. wet room
    d. blanket wrap ____

30. How often should you mix a new batch of herbs with water in the heating unit, ideally?
    a. twice every day
    b. twice every week
    c. once every day
    d. once every week   ____

31. What should you use to retrieve linens or wraps from the heating unit?
    a. bare hands
    b. cotton swabs
    c. plastic spatula
    d. rubber-gloved hands   ____

32. How long should an herbal wrap process on the client's body?
    a. 30 minutes
    b. 45 minutes
    c. one hour
    d. 90 minutes   ____

33. How hot should the water in the heating unit be when you insert the muslin pouch filled with water-soluble herbs, when preparing for an herbal wrap?
    a. 105°F
    b. 165°F
    c. 205°F
    d. 265°F   ____

34. Why is linen the preferred material for herbal wraps?
    a. it has a softer texture than other materials
    b. it has a more attractive appearance than other materials
    c. it maintains heat longer than other materials
    d. it absorbs moisture better than other materials   ____

35. What function does walnut leaf powder serve in an herbal scrub?
    a. moisturizing
    b. soothing
    c. skin cell regeneration
    d. cleansing   ____

CHAPTER 22—COMPLEMENTARY WELLNESS THERAPIES

1. When did humans come to view themselves as separate from nature?
   a. Industrial Age
   b. Renaissance
   c. Middle Ages
   d. Colonial Era
   _____

2. How many classifications with complementary and alternative medicine (CAM) are recognized by the National Institutes of Health (NIH)?
   a. three
   b. five
   c. seven
   d. nine
   _____

3. What is the basis for everything and is found in humans, animals, nature, and objects?
   a. water
   b. air
   c. energy
   d. matter
   _____

4. How do you feel when you are full of energy?
   a. ill and stressed
   b. healthy and stressed
   c. ill and vibrant
   d. healthy and vibrant
   _____

5. How do you feel when you lack energy?
   a. ill and stressed
   b. ill and vibrant
   c. healthy and vibrant
   d. healthy and stressed
   _____

6. What happens to our subtle body energy bodies as we grow up?
   a. they mature into full strength
   b. they are diminished by negativity
   c. they disappear as we enter adulthood
   d. they emerge as we enter adulthood
   _____

7. How far from the body does the energy bubble known as one's aura extend?
   a. 3 to 5 feet
   b. indefinitely
   c. 1 to 12 inches
   d. less than 1 inch
   _____

8. When do you represent your authentic self and exhibit what would be labeled as your "good" qualities?
   a. when you work with others
   b. when you work alone
   c. whenever you are awake and alert
   d. when you are in balance
   _____

9. When do you exhibit what would be labeled as your "bad" qualities?
   a. when you are out of balance
   b. whenever you are awake and alert
   c. when you work with others
   d. when you work alone   ____

10. What do photographs taken with Kirilan cameras reveal?
    a. patches of dry skin   c. large deposits of fat
    b. colors of the aura   d. internal toxins   ____

11. What term refers to a methodology used to balance all aspects of body, mind, and spirit?
    a. wellness management   c. energy management
    b. wellness organization   d. energy organization   ____

12. What does **NOT** throw you off balance?
    a. alcohol   c. prescription drugs
    b. tobacco   d. relaxation   ____

13. What term refers to your outlook on life and reactions to daily events, based upon the information your brain receives and processes?
    a. cognitive intelligence   c. spirit intelligence
    b. emotional intelligence   d. energy intelligence   ____

14. What gives you the ability to tell the difference between who you *are* and who others *want* you to be?
    a. mental body   c. spirit/energy body
    b. emotional body   d. physical body   ____

15. What ancient culture believed that the soul, or psyche, was responsible for one's behavior?
    a. Japanese   c. Greeks
    b. Chinese   d. Egyptians   ____

16. What are also called herbal tinctures?
    a. capsules   c. tablets
    b. herbal teas   d. herbal elixirs   ____

17. What is **NOT** an example of a rebalancing breathing exercise?
    a. breathe in limitations and breathe out abundance
    b. breathe in acceptance and breathe out judgments
    c. breathe in confidence and breathe out doubt
    d. breathe in peacefulness and breathe out anxiety   ____

126

18. What is the meaning of the Sanskrit word from which the word *chakra* is derived?
    a. wheel of balance
    b. wheel of light
    c. circle of balance
    d. circle of light

    _____

19. What chakras are related to the development of conscious awareness?
    a. only the first chakra
    b. chakras one through three
    c. chakras four through seven
    d. only the seventh chakra

    _____

20. What chakra is associated with the right eye?
    a. fourth
    b. fifth
    c. sixth
    d. seventh

    _____

21. What chakra is associated with the left eye?
    a. fourth
    b. fifth
    c. sixth
    d. seventh

    _____

22. What is the nature of the sixth chakra?
    a. holistic mind/visionary
    b. intuitive intelligence
    c. individuality, sense of purpose
    d. concrete mind

    _____

23. What is the nature of the second chakra?
    a. male energy
    b. female energy
    c. individuality, sense of purpose
    d. holistic mind, visionary

    _____

24. What chakra is related to the female reproductive organs?
    a. fifth
    b. fourth
    c. third
    d. second

    _____

25. How do you become the example that others want to follow?
    a. by improving yourself
    b. by calling yourself a healer
    c. by offering wellness modalities
    d. by adding Reiki to your service menu

    _____

26. What statement about Reiki is correct?
    a. you can receive other people's negative energy when you perform it
    b. it works to heal the cause of imbalance and eliminate it
    c. it should not be performed on people who are taking blood thinners
    d. it should not be combined with any other therapeutic or healing technique _____

27. How long after receiving first-level Reiki attunements should you wait before receiving second-level Reiki attunements?
    a. two hours   c. two weeks
    b. two days   d. two months _____

28. How long after receiving your second-level Reiki attunements should you practice consistently on yourself before going to the Reiki master level?
    a. at least three months   c. at least three years
    b. at least six months   d. at least six years _____

29. How long does a person stay attuned to Reiki?
    a. a few hours   c. up to a year
    b. several weeks   d. for life _____

30. What natural objects are the focus of remedies developed by Dr. Edward Bach?
    a. stones   c. crystals
    b. flowers   d. soils _____

31. What is the therapeutic benefit of the white chestnut flower essence?
    a. helping set boundaries and providing protection from outside sources
    b. finding a middle ground for those who tend to go to extremes
    c. reducing mental chatter and providing mental clarity
    d. healing emotional wounds and encouraging acceptance _____

32. What is the therapeutic benefit of the holly flower essence?
    a. reducing mental chatter and providing mental clarity
    b. helping set boundaries and providing protection from outside sources
    c. finding a middle ground for those who tend to go to extremes
    d. healing emotional wounds and encouraging acceptance _____

33. What term refers to products that have been attuned energetically with universal healing energy?
    a. energy infusions
    c. crystals
    b. Reiki attunements
    d. gemstones _____

34. What ancient culture used crystal gazing to induce altered states of mind to receive spirit messages and see into the future?
    a. Greeks
    c. Chinese
    b. Egyptians
    d. Japanese _____

35. What color is energizing and helps lift the spirits?
    a. green
    c. yellow
    b. red
    d. blue _____

CHAPTER 23—AYURVEDA THEORY AND TREATMENTS

1. What is a benefit of learning the marma points?
   a. deepens the relaxation your clients' experience
   b. cures chronic medical conditions
   c. makes treatments more exciting and stimulating
   d. improves clients' muscle tone ____

2. What practice is **NOT** derived from Ayurveda?
   a. foot reflexology   c. full-body oil massage
   b. heat therapy   d. kinesiology ____

3. What condition is caused by an excess of the element earth?
   a. puffiness or edema   c. cellulite
   b. redness or inflammation d. osteoporosis ____

4. What does the word *vata* mean?
   a. to heat or burn   c. to move or enthuse
   b. to embrace or keep together d. to yoke or unite ____

5. What is an example of the open quality of the element space?
   a. fidgety, talkative client
   b. client who is open-minded
   c. client with soft, moist skin
   d. client with firm skin that ages well ____

6. What term refers to the ancient writing of the rishis, the Indian mystics who first recorded Ayurveda?
   a. Mantra   c. Vedas
   b. Pitta Dosha   d. Purvakarma ____

7. What condition is caused by an excess of the element water?
   a. osteoporosis
   b. cellulite
   c. redness or inflammation
   d. puffiness or edema ____

8. What makes up a human being, according to Ayurveda?
   a. bone, fiber, and tissue
   b. a interconnected network of muscles, organs, systems, and tissues
   c. air and water
   d. an ever-changing, dynamic collection of energy and intelligence ____

9. What is the focus of Ayurvedic Principle and Application No. 1?
   a. the six-sense approach
   b. moving clients toward goals
   c. working with the three doshas
   d. carefully selected products ____

10. What sense is affected by things like voices and music?
   a. sight   c. hearing
   b. smell   d. touch ____

11. What sense is affected by aromatherapy?
   a. taste   c. sight
   b. touch   d. smell ____

12. What dosha is dominant in a client who is slender, small, and light-boned with light musculature?
   a. kapha   c. amalki
   b. pitta   d. vata ____

13. What is an example of the inspirational quality of the element air?
   a. the client whose skin flares up and who complains about stuffy rooms
   b. an open-minded client
   c. the staff member whose presence feels like a breath of fresh air
   d. someone who handles difficulties well ____

14. What Ayurvedic Principle and Application involves using a caring attitude to notice details of the client's physical being, like body frame and facial structure?
   a. Principle and Application No. 2
   b. Principle and Application No. 3
   c. Principle and Application No. 4
   d. Principle and Application No. 5 ____

15. What condition is caused by an excess of the element fire?
   a. redness or inflammation   c. osteoporosis
   b. puffiness or edema   d. cellulite ____

16. What term refers to the five great elements that come together the second a person is conceived?
   a. purvakarmas   c. shirodhras
   b. panchamahabhutas   d. doshas ____

17. What should Ayurvedic beauty and personal-care products provide?
    a. a glamorous look
    b. chemical stimulants
    c. needed nutrients for the skin
    d. a sexually alluring fragrance   _____

18. What is **NOT** a common ingredient for Ayurvedic beauty and
    personal-care products?
    a. organic, cold-pressed oils
    b. dried herbs
    c. flower petals
    d. scientifically engineered compounds   _____

19. What dosha is dominant in a client who has a medium build and
    good posture and who is athletic and well-balanced?
    a. pitta   c. vata
    b. amalki   d. kapha   _____

20. What term refers to a blend of the three doshas?
    a. constitutional body-mind type
    b. Ayurvedic body-mind type
    c. constitutional mind-body blend
    d. Ayurvedic mind-body blend   _____

21. What is **NOT** true about doshas?
    a. they are vibrational modes in subatomic matter
    b. they can be measured by scientific instruments
    c. we experience them in the rhythms of nature
    d. they naturally tend to change, move, and become unbalanced   _____

22. What condition is caused by an excess of the element air?
    a. redness or inflammation   c. osteoporosis
    b. dryness or flaking   d. cellulite   _____

23. What does the word "pitta" mean?
    a. to move or enthuse
    b. to yoke or unite
    c. to embrace or keep together
    d. to heat or burn   _____

24. What is an example of the upward-moving quality of the element fire?
    a. a regular client who loves time-proven treatments
    b. someone who handles difficulties well
    c. someone whose skin is cold to the touch or has cold hands
    d. someone with tremendous ambition   ____

25. What is an example of the lubricating quality of the element water?
    a. someone who handles difficulties well
    b. a fidgety, talkative client
    c. someone with tremendous ambition
    d. a client with firm skin that ages well   ____

26. What condition is caused by an excess of the element space?
    a. cellulite   c. osteoporosis
    b. dryness or flaking   d. puffiness or edema   ____

27. What dosha is dominant in a client who has a strong build with square or rounded shapes and who is heavy-boned and well proportioned?
    a. amalki   c. pitta
    b. kapha   d. vata   ____

28. What is the focus of Ayurvedic Principle and Application No. 5?
    a. working with the three doshas
    b. carefully selecting products
    c. the six-sense approach
    d. moving clients toward goals   ____

29. How many major marma points are used in full-body therapeutic sequences?
    a. 17   c. 107
    b. 71   d. 1,007   ____

30. What effect can stress have on marma points?
    a. relocating them   c. creating them
    b. activating them   d. closing them   ____

31. What is a major common way to open marma points?
    a. gentle touch   c. enzyme peels
    b. vigorous massage   d. microcurrent   ____

32. What is an example of the stable quality of the element earth?
    a. a client who is eager to try new things
    b. a regular client who loves time-proven treatments
    c. someone with tremendous ambition
    d. the staff member whose presence feels like a breath of fresh air ____

33. What does the word *kapha* mean?
    a. to embrace or keep together   c. to yoke or unite
    b. to heat or burn   d. to move or enthuse ____

34. What is **NOT** true of a client's state of being when his or her marma points are open and healthy?
    a. the needs of the skin are well met
    b. the client's skin is dull and flat
    c. the client feels good inside
    d. the client's mind is relaxed ____

35. Where on the face should marma massage be applied in order to relieve jaw tension?
    a. top of the neck   c. root of the ear
    b. eyes   d. joints in the skull ____

Part 6: Medical Sciences

CHAPTER 24—WORKING IN A MEDICAL SETTING

1. What is a common obstacle to advancement facing outsiders working at family-run businesses?
    a. nepotism
    b. sexism
    c. ageism
    d. racism

    A

2. What is a true of a top-down human resource methodology?
    a. ideas are introduced by the boss and then discussed with the staff
    b. control and direction come only from the person in charge
    c. the senior person is laid off first during economic downturns
    d. workers are encouraged to criticize the decisions of management

    B

3. How should you regard the people who seek treatment in a medical setting?
    a. customers
    b. partners
    c. patients
    d. clients

    C

4. What is a top priority at all times in the medical setting?
    a. keeping the mood light
    b. generating retail sales
    c. generating conversation
    d. maintaining confidentiality

    D

5. What attitude toward fraternization is common in the medical setting?
    a. this represents an unacceptable crossing of professional boundaries
    b. the office should be as silent as a library at all times
    c. chatting with coworkers during business hours is encouraged
    d. chatting with patients during procedures is encouraged

    A

6. Who is **NOT** among the professionals with whom medical charts are frequently shared?
    a. physicians
    b. prospective patients
    c. lawyers
    d. insurance agents

    B

7. What should an esthetician who wishes to integrate seamlessly into the medical esthetic practice understand?
    a. medical billing
    b. legal billing
    c. medical terminology
    d. legal terminology

    _C_

8. What is **NOT** something that is evaluated using the scientific method?
    a. drugs
    b. procedures
    c. equipment
    d. personnel

    _D_

9. What term refers to the difference between the results experienced by a control group and the results experienced by an experimental group?
    a. statistical significance
    b. statistical difference
    c. scientific significance
    d. scientific difference

    _A_

10. How many steps are there in the scientific method?
    a. three
    b. five
    c. seven
    d. nine

    _B_

11. When was the Federal Packaging and Labeling Act, which requires cosmetic manufacturers to list ingredients, voted into law?
    a. 1917
    b. 1947
    c. 1977
    d. 2007

    _C_

12. How can you earn greater support and trust while interfacing with medical professionals?
    a. by declaring that you already know everything you need to know
    b. by demonstrating that you work best alone, without supervision
    c. by declaring that learning about medicine is not part of your job
    d. by demonstrating that you are open to learning as much as you can

    _D_

13. What do you do when you adopt the same core values and work approaches that the medical team presents?
    a. support the medical team
    b. join the medical team
    c. substitute for the medical team
    d. eliminate the need for the medical team

    _A_

14. What should you share with new staff members?
    a. your opinions of coworkers' skills
    b. your knowledge of office-wide protocols
    c. private information about patients
    d. private information about salaries

    _B_

15. What should you offer to your team members when integrating new products and/or treatments?
    a. liability disclaimers   c. in-service training
    b. scientific analyses   d. free services

    _C_

16. What should you do if the medical staff in your office is required to attend a seminar?
    a. schedule a vacation day
    b. meet private clients at home to make some extra money
    c. attend the seminar if possible
    d. schedule an office party to keep up workplace morale

    _C_

17. What is it imperative that estheticians working in a medical setting obtain?
    a. medical degrees   c. psychological counseling
    b. liability insurance   d. continuing education

    _D_

18. What title does a nurse with a four-year college nursing education traditionally receive?
    a. registered nurse   c. doctor of medicine
    b. licensed practical nurse   d. physician's assistant

    _A_

19. What title does a nurse with a two-year college nursing education traditionally receive?
    a. physician's assistant   c. registered nurse
    b. licensed practical nurse   d. doctor of medicine

    _B_

20. How many total years of post-high school education are usually required for students to receive a master's degree?
    a. two   c. six
    b. four   d. eight

    _C_

21. How many years of education do physicians generally receive beyond high school?
    a. two   c. six
    b. four   d. eight

    _D_

22. Who must supervise the work in a medical spa according to the definition provided by the National Coalition of Estheticians, Manufacturers/Distributors & Associations?
    a. highly trained esthetician
    b. licensed health care professional
    c. experienced salon manager
    d. licensed dermatologist

    _B_

23. What term refers to physicians who specialize in performing surgery for cosmetic or reconstructive purposes?
    a. skin care specialists
    c. plastic surgeons
    b. estheticians
    d. dermatologists

    c

24. What type of surgical procedures are generally associated with cosmetic plastic surgeons?
    a. reconstructive
    c. cardiological
    b. emergency
    d. elective

    D

25. What is **NOT** an example of an elective surgical procedure?
    a. cleft lip correction
    c. face lift
    b. eye lift
    d. breast augmentation

    A

26. What type of surgery is **NOT** associated with reconstructive surgeons?
    a. cleft lip correction
    b. breast augmentation
    c. removal of skin-cancer lesion
    d. repair following an accident

    B

27. What term refers to a subspecialty of dermatology that treats appearance-related skin conditions, such as wrinkles, scars, hyperpigmentation, and hyperplasia?
    a. cosmetic surgery
    c. cosmetic dermatology
    b. esthetic surgery
    d. esthetic dermatology

    C

28. What is **NOT** among the reasons physicians have recently entered the esthetics field in greater numbers than before?
    a. financial opportunity
    c. financial constraints of managed care
    b. advances in technology
    d. decreased credibility for physicians

    D

29. What is the best source of information if you have a question about state regulations with regard to your scope of practice?
    a. state licensing board
    b. salon bulletin board
    c. Internet chat rooms
    d. word of mouth among coworkers

    A

30. What role sometimes blurs with the role the esthetician plays in a medical setting?
    a. surgeon
    c. registered nurse
    b. medical assistant
    d. licensed practical nurse

    B

31. What is the average number of hours of training required before an esthetician can be licensed?
    a. 150
    b. 300
    c. 600
    d. 950

    C

32. What is **NOT** among the changes that many are demanding because of the current state of esthetic licensing requirements?
    a. increased education
    b. more progressive regulations
    c. national standards
    d. looser definitions

    D

33. What is a new form of licensure now recognized in Utah, Virginia, and the District of Columbia?
    a. master esthetician
    b. medical esthetician
    c. master skin care specialist
    d. medical skin care specialist

    A

34. What title have some estheticians with a results-oriented/scientific focus chosen to use even though it is not officially recognized?
    a. registered esthetician
    b. clinical esthetician
    c. practical esthetician
    d. surgical esthetician

    B

35. What is a primary factor in developing a dual relationship between the practice and the patient?
    a. hard selling
    b. soft selling
    c. trust
    d. friendship

    C

CHAPTER 25—MEDICAL TERMINOLOGY

1. What document that is critical for proper client care can only be understood by people with knowledge of medical terminology?
    a. client's medical record
    b. salon intake form
    c. patient billing invoice
    d. pharmaceutical prescription ____

2. What part of the word "dermatology" is the suffix?
    a. "dermat"   c. "matol"
    b. "ology"   d. "derm" ____

3. What is the meaning of the prefix "ante," as in the word "antemortem"?
    a. multiple   c. before
    b. cancerous   d. contagious ____

4. What does the Latin root "bull" mean?
    a. blister   c. hair
    b. hardened skin   d. cancer ____

5. What sound is made by the letter combination "ph," as in "phrenoplegia"?
    a. f   c. k
    b. r   d. dis ____

6. What is a way for remembering eponyms?
    a. utilizing pneumonic devices
    b. all eponyms have the same prefix
    c. all eponyms have the same suffix
    d. repeated exposure to the words ____

7. What Latin root means "nostril"?
    a. mal   c. nar
    b. ocul   d. nerv ____

8. What is the meaning of the Greek prefix "dys," as in "dystrophy"?
    a. sweet   c. good
    b. sour   d. bad ____

9. Who recognized the need for a universal language of medicine?
    a. Hippocrates   c. Homer
    b. Imhotep   d. Tutankhamen ____

10. What does the Greek root "blephar" mean?
    a. toenail   c. nipple
    b. eyelid   d. fingernail   _____

11. When a singular medical term ends in "is," as in "diagnosis," what
    should you generally replace "is" with in order to form the plural of
    the medical term?
    a. "es"   c. "i"
    b. "a"   d. "ae"   _____

12. What does the Greek root "hist" mean?
    a. tissue   c. muscle
    b. bone   d. skin   _____

13. What is an example of a medical term from the Middle Ages that is
    now considered politically incorrect?
    a. cleft chin   c. Adam's apple
    b. clubfoot   d. Achilles' heel   _____

14. What is the meaning of the Greek prefix "peri," as in "peripheral"?
    a. around   c. more
    b. before   d. less   _____

15. What does the Greek root "hem" mean?
    a. sebum   c. blood
    b. sweat   d. lymph   _____

16. When did maritime advancements in shipbuilding and cartography
    allow more extensive travel, leading to an intercontinental influence
    in medical terminology?
    a. Paleolithic Era   c. Renaissance
    b. Middle Ages   d. Industrial Age   _____

17. What is true about words within the realm of medical technology
    that carry judgment or reflect opinions toward affected populations?
    a. no such words exist within the realm of medical terminology
    b. these words cannot be changed because of their longtime use
    c. all of these words have been successfully eliminated
    d. elimination of these words is a chief goal of modern terminology   _____

18. Where does understanding medical terminology begin?
    a. analysis   c. pluralization
    b. pronunciation   d. spelling   _____

19. What does the Greek root "derm" mean?
    a. tissue   c. bone
    b. muscle   d. skin   _____

20. What Greek root means "disease"?
    a. path   c. phot
    b. plast   d. phleb   _____

21. What does the Greek prefix "hypo" mean, as in "hypophrenia"?
    a. above   c. under
    b. less   d. more   _____

22. What sound is made by the letter combination "ch," as in "cochlea"?
    a. ch   c. r
    b. k   d. z   _____

23. What is an example of a combining vowel?
    a. a "y" at the end of a word
    b. an "o" in the middle of a word
    c. an "a" at the end of the word
    d. a "c" in the middle of a word   _____

24. What term refers to the union of a root word and a combining vowel?
    a. modifying form   c. combining form
    b. modifying terminology   d. combining terminology _____

25. What part of the word "dermatology" is the prefix?
    a. the word does not have a prefix   c. "dermat"
    b. "matol"   d. "ology"   _____

26. What term refers to qualifying or limiting the meaning of a word?
    a. combine   c. suffix
    b. prefix   d. modify   _____

27. When a singular medical term ends in "a," as in "vertebra," what should you generally replace the "a" with in order to form the plural of the medical term?
    a. "um"   c. "ina"
    b. "ae"   d. "ces"   _____

28. What Greek root means "dark"?
    a. morph   c. ophthalm
    b. necr   d. melan   _____

29. What does the Latin prefix "retro" mean, as in "retronasal"?
    a. again   c. backward
    b. somewhat   d. through   _____

30. What is true about some words ending in "-ix" or "-ax"?
    a. these words are already plural and need no further modification
    b. they cannot be made into plurals
    c. they have more than one acceptable plural form
    d. they are not used in medicine   _____

31. What does the Greek root "lip" mean?
    a. lymph   c. blood
    b. fat   d. red   _____

32. What roots can be found in the word "matrilineal"?
    a. "matri" and "neal"   c. "mat" and "neal"
    b. "lin" and "eal"   d. "matri" and "lineal" _____

33. What Greek root means "poison"?
    a. troph   c. trich
    b. tox   d. therm   _____

34. What does the Latin prefix "ultra" mean, as in "ultrasound"?
    a. away   c. across
    b. behind   d. beyond   _____

35. What sound is made by the letter "x" in a medical term such as "xanthic"?
    a. f   c. z
    b. k   d. r   _____

CHAPTER 26—MEDICAL INTERVENTION

1. What led to the creation of the multibillion-dollar industry called nonsurgical esthetics?
   a. public desire to fight visible signs of aging
   b. public desire to arrest dangerous skin diseases
   c. widespread trend toward the use of permanent makeup
   d. widespread trend toward the use of spray tanning _____

2. What is typically the esthetician's role in vein therapy?
   a. performing the procedure
   b. answering questions
   c. making medical recommendations
   d. removing sutures _____

3. What service falls within the field of esthetics, as opposed to the field of medical esthetics?
   a. Botox Cosmetic
   b. dermal fillers
   c. microdermabrasion
   d. injection vein therapy _____

4. Why must you be vigilant about updating information you give to clients and checking its accuracy?
   a. your advice is considered a legally binding contract
   b. your advice is considered an official medical diagnosis
   c. lawsuits regularly make once-popular products illegal
   d. new products come into the market regularly _____

5. What is **NOT** an example of the general information you can share with a client without consequences?
   a. diagnosis of medical condition
   b. information about types of products
   c. information about product durability
   d. what to expect in postcare _____

6. When should you make endorsements for particular products?
   a. if you have used the product
   b. never
   c. sometimes
   d. if you trust the manufacturer _____

7. What government agency approves the pharmaceuticals used in medical esthetics?
   a. United States Department of Agriculture (USDA)
   b. Food and Drug Administration (FDA)
   c. Occupational Safety and Health Administration (OSHA)
   d. Centers for Disease Control and Prevention (CDC)   ____

8. What is **NOT** a factor in determining product durability?
   a. type of material used   c. cost of the service
   b. location of the placement   d. depth of the placement   ____

9. What term refers to dynamic wrinkles that connect the nose to the mouth?
   a. necrosis   c. platysmal bands
   b. strabismus   d. nasolabial lines   ____

10. What is the bacterium from which Botox Cosmetic and Dysport are derived?
    a. botulinum toxin   c. mycobacterium leprae
    b. bordetella pertusssis   d. neisseria gonorrhoeae   ____

11. How long will the original result that is achieved with dermal fillers, the result from a client's first injection session, last?
    a. one to two months
    b. four to eight months
    c. nine months to one year
    d. one to two years   ____

12. What is **NOT** among the key ingredients for youthful-looking skin?
    a. hyaluronic acid   c. elastin
    b. collagen   d. neurotoxin   ____

13. What term refers to movement caused by active motion of muscles and nerve tissue?
    a. active movement   c. active motion
    b. dynamic movement   d. dynamic motion   ____

14. What term refers to a situation that occurs when a needle is inserted into a blood vessel and a drop of filler material occludes the blood flow to the skin, causing the skin to die?
    a. nasolabial lines   c. necrosis
    b. platysmal bands   d. strabismus   ____

15. What happens if product is placed more deeply than is recommended?
    a. it will lose all efficacy
    b. it will cause an itchy rash
    c. it will infect the bloodstream
    d. it will absorb more quickly ____

16. What is **NOT** among the desirable qualities for a perfect injectable material?
    a. extensive product migration
    b. forgiving in placement
    c. hypoallergenic
    d. few side effects ____

17. What is the result of injecting a product like Prevelle Silk into the midpapillary dermis, rather than the intended injection site of the upper epidermis?
    a. the product's effect wears off quickly
    b. the product's effect is permanent
    c. the client develops an allergy to the product
    d. the product loses all efficacy ____

18. How long after the first injection of dermal filler will material reside in the tissues?
    a. up to one week
    b. up to one month
    c. one year or more
    d. permanently ____

19. Why do follow-up injections of product, taking place six months after the original treatment, deliver longer-lasting results?
    a. the skin has produced substantial amounts of new collagen
    b. the skin has produced substantial amounts of new elastin
    c. the client has developed a tolerance
    d. the new product is added to a foundation ____

20. What is **NOT** among the common indications for neurotoxins?
    a. high cheekbones
    b. frown lines
    c. crow's feet
    d. chin pebbling ____

21. What is a good response when clients ask about the durability of a specific neurotoxin?
    a. one to two months
    b. three to five months
    c. seven to nine months
    d. about one year ____

22. How long is the typical treatment time for a Botox Cosmetic or Dysport injection session?
    a. three hours
    b. one hour
    c. 15 minutes
    d. five minutes ____

23. What can clients who request full paralysis from a neurotoxin treatment expect?
    a. more visible results
    b. less visible results
    c. more longevity of results
    d. less longevity of results ____

24. Where on the face can a careless product injection lead to eyelid ptosis?
    a. eyebrow
    b. upper cheek
    c. lower forehead
    d. upper forehead ____

25. When should you make recommendations about medical procedures?
    a. if you've had the procedure
    b. sometimes
    c. never
    d. if you trust a particular physician ____

26. What is **NOT** among the treatment results that Botox Cosmetic delivers?
    a. erasing fine lines
    b. improving facial contour
    c. addressing eye shape
    d. permanently correcting conditions ____

27. What allergy is a contraindication for Dysport injections?
    a. allergy to cow's milk
    b. lactose intolerance
    c. hay fever
    d. allergy to peanuts ____

28. What does a black box warning, found on products including Botox Cosmetic and Dysport, state?
    a. black bruises will occur after product injection
    b. death can occur if product reaches unintended areas
    c. use of the product includes a high fatality rate
    d. repeated use of the product will cause death ____

29. How frequently must clients sign consent forms for the use of neurotoxins?
    a. only at the first visit
    b. never
    c. each visit
    d. once per year ____

30. What is **NOT** among the indications for dermal fillers?
    a. hollow cheeks
    c. weak chin
    b. rosacea
    d. deep winkles and creases   ____

31. What are dermal fillers sometimes called?
    a. liquid dermabrasion
    c. liquid face-lifts
    b. chemical dermabrasion
    d. chemical face-lifts   ____

32. Where in the body does hyaluronic acid operate as a lubricant and a shock absorber?
    a. muscles
    c. organs
    b. capillaries
    d. joints   ____

33. What product has been approved by the FDA?
    a. Juvederm
    c. Dermalive
    b. Macrolane
    d. Viscontour   ____

34. What is left after necrosis heals?
    a. hyperpigmented lesion
    c. pockmark
    b. scar
    d. stretch mark   ____

35. What is the key to successful outcomes?
    a. pricing
    c. communication
    b. scheduling
    d. speed   ____

CHAPTER 27—PLASTIC SURGERY PROCEDURES

1. Where on the body are the circumareolar areas found?
   a. breasts
   c. cheeks
   b. buttocks
   d. thighs _____

2. What term refers to the use of an electrical device to cut the skin or to seal blood vessels to control bleeding during surgery?
   a. electrotherapy
   c. electrolysis
   b. electrocautery
   d. electrocution _____

3. What is the medical term for a breast lift procedure?
   a. mammoplasty
   c. mastopexy
   b. mammography
   d. mastectomy _____

4. What is **NOT** true of the nasal turbinates?
   a. they are areas of bone and mucosa
   b. they protrude from the lateral walls of the nasal cavity
   c. they can sometimes cause nasal airway obstruction
   d. they dry inhaled air _____

5. What term refers to the area within the anatomic triangular margins of the mandible where the double chin resides?
   a. submental
   c. nasolabial
   b. periorbital
   d. endonasal _____

6. What is **NOT** among the reasons "baby boomers" have embraced plastic surgery?
   a. they are living longer
   b. surgery costs have decreased significantly
   c. they have higher disposable income
   d. they are less tolerant of aging _____

7. Why is it important to be knowledgeable about medical skin procedures?
   a. because estheticians are expected to perform the medical consultation
   b. because estheticians are expected to participate in all of these procedures
   c. to help you recommend proper post-treatment services
   d. to identify the procedures that should be performed _____

8. What is **NOT** true about the patient's experience under local anesthesia?
   a. the patient may feel some tugging
   b. the patient feels very little pain
   c. the patient is relaxed
   d. the patient is asleep ____

9. What is **NOT** among the factors that dictate the anesthesia method used?
   a. cost of the procedure
   c. extent of the procedure
   b. patient's health
   d. physician's preference ____

10. What part of the face is **LEAST** affected by a rhytidectomy?
    a. cheeks
    c. jawline
    b. forehead
    d. mouth/nose area ____

11. What procedure works best on superficial lines and wrinkles, pigmentation, and irregularities?
    a. rhytidectomy
    c. resurfacing
    b. blepharoplasty
    d. facial liposuction ____

12. What is the age range of most face-lift patients?
    a. teens to twenties
    c. twenties to forties
    b. eighties and older
    d. forties to sixties ____

13. How far in advance of a rhytidectomy procedure must the patient stop smoking?
    a. one to two days
    c. three to four weeks
    b. one to two weeks
    d. three to four months ____

14. What is the worst-case scenario if a patient smokes before surgery?
    a. hyperpigmentation
    c. hypopigmentation
    b. necrosis
    d. discomfort ____

15. What differentiates the various rhytidectomy techniques?
    a. age of the patient
    c. depth of the dissection plane
    b. skin color of the patient
    d. type of anesthesia used ____

16. What should be applied to the surgery area for 48 hours after a thread lift?
    a. concealing makeup
    c. heating pad
    b. gentle massage
    d. ice compresses ____

17. What part of the face is affected by a brow lift?
    a. upper third
    b. upper two-thirds
    c. middle third
    d. lower third
    _____

18. Why do some patients receiving a brow lift also receive concomitant skin resurfacing, a face-lift, and/or a blepharoplasty?
    a. to minimize the side effects of the brow lift
    b. to improve overall texture of the skin
    c. because a brow lift cannot be performed as a stand-alone service
    d. to prepare for a later collagen injection procedure
    _____

19. What surgery might a patient with significant overhang of the upper eyelids consider adding to a forehead lift procedure?
    a. mastoplasty
    b. open rhinoplasty
    c. blepharoplasty
    d. closed rhinoplasty
    _____

20. What is a benefit of an endoscopic forehead lift as opposed to a classic forehead lift?
    a. less excision of muscle
    b. more dramatic results
    c. longer-lasting results
    d. quicker recovery
    _____

21. What is **NOT** among the factors the surgeon considers while deciding on the placement of incisions prior to performing a forehead lift?
    a. weight of the patient
    b. facial structure
    c. condition of the skin
    d. placement of the hairline
    _____

22. Where is the coronal incision made during a forehead lift?
    a. across the top of the skull
    b. slightly behind the natural hairline
    c. across the base of the skull
    d. along the line of the eyebrows
    _____

23. How long do most forehead lift procedures take?
    a. 20 to 30 minutes
    b. 30 minutes to one hour
    c. one to two hours
    d. two to four hours
    _____

24. What is **NOT** among the medical conditions that make blepharoplasty riskier than usual?
    a. Graves' disease
    b. a lack of sufficient tears
    c. hypothyroidism
    d. photophobia
    _____

25. What is **NOT** among the places where blepharoplasty can be performed?
    a. beauty salon
    b. surgeon's office-based facility
    c. outpatient surgery center
    d. hospital
    _____

26. What treatment might a patient with excess wrinkles below the eyes consider adding to a blepharoplasty procedure?
    a. microdermabrasion
    b. open rhinoplasty
    c. laser resurfacing
    d. closed rhinoplasty
    _____

27. How many days should a patient wait following blepharoplasty before showering?
    a. one to two
    b. three to four
    c. six to eight
    d. at least 10
    _____

28. What is the goal of cosmetic rhinoplasty?
    a. to make the nose the most prominent feature of the face
    b. to address medical problems like a deviated nasal septum
    c. to shift the nose to a higher position on the face
    d. to create harmony between the nose and other facial features
    _____

29. Why do most surgeons prefer to delay operating on younger patients?
    a. to wait for the patients to complete their growth spurts
    b. to avoid costly litigation
    c. to wait for patients to reach the age of legal consent
    d. to avoid irritating teen acne
    _____

30. What is **NOT** among the preprocedure considerations for rhinoplasty?
    a. shape of the septum
    b. amount of periorbital fat
    c. thickness of the skin
    d. patient's age and race
    _____

31. What medical condition might be a contraindication for facial implants?
    a. asthma
    b. acne
    c. gum disease
    d. hirsutism
    _____

32. How long might insertion of a chin implant take?
    a. three to four hours
    b. 90 minutes to two hours
    c. one hour to 90 minutes
    d. 30 minutes to one hour
    _____

33. What effect do breast implants have on the patient's fertility, according to current evidence?
    a. fertility is not affected
    b. fertility is temporarily diminished
    c. fertility is permanently diminished
    d. they cause infertility _____

34. What surgery might a patient with sagging breasts consider adding to a breast augmentation procedure?
    a. liposuction
    b. mastopexy
    c. blepharoplasty
    d. mastectomy _____

35. Why should patients who are planning to lose a significant amount of weight and/or become pregnant consider postponing breast implant surgery?
    a. either event will greatly diminish the size of the patient's breasts
    b. either event will reverse the effects of breast implant surgery
    c. these events can alter breast size in an unpredictable manner
    d. these events can lead to implant-related infections _____

CHAPTER 28—THE ESTHETICIAN'S ROLE IN PRE- AND POST-MEDICAL TREATMENTS

1. When can you help clients adhere to medical intervention guidelines to minimize the risk of infection and maximize the client's outcome?
   a. after a laser procedure
   b. during a laser procedure
   c. a few weeks before a laser procedure
   d. a few months before a laser procedure ____

2. Who is responsible for recommending therapeutic products for home use, organizing a home care program, and explaining the importance of these products to the client?
   a. physician   c. medical assistant
   b. esthetician   d. nurse ____

3. What term is **MOST** appropriate when speaking with medical professionals regarding a person under their care?
   a. patron   c. patient
   b. customer   d. client ____

4. What term is most appropriate when speaking about a person who is **NOT** under a physician's care but instead comes to your place of business for esthetic services?
   a. patron   c. patient
   b. customer   d. client ____

5. What purpose do amino acids, green tea, hyaluronic acids, and vitamins C and E serve in presurgery home care kits?
   a. moisturization   c. exfoliation
   b. cleansing   d. sun protection ____

6. When do you have opportunities to counsel the client on the importance of postprocedure skin care and long-term skin maintenance?
   a. premedical and/or laser treatments
   b. initial client consultations
   c. initial postsurgical treatments
   d. therapeutic massage sessions ____

7. What is **NOT** among the factors considered when designing a treatment plan?
   a. patient's skin type   c. physician protocol
   b. patient's sexual activity   d. level of photo-aging ____

8. What do classic cleansing facials, enzyme peels, microcurrent facial toning, microdermabrasion, and ultrasonic treatments have in common?
   a. they all require anesthesia
   b. they must be performed by physicians
   c. they can be performed in-office
   d. they have high risk factors _____

9. What is an appropriate response when a client says he or she is anxious about an upcoming procedure?
   a. suggest canceling the procedure
   b. inform the client that preprocedure anxiety is abnormal
   c. suggest delaying the procedure
   d. recommend conveying those concerns to the doctor _____

10. When is it acceptable to use acids stronger than normally allowed by your scope of practice?
   a. when you are working under a physician's supervision
   b. when you have client consent
   c. when you are working under the salon manager's supervision
   d. at any time _____

11. When must you be especially careful about performing microdermabrasion?
   a. when the client has cancer
   b. when the client has rosacea
   c. when the client is very thin
   d. when the client is obese _____

12. How do enzymes such as bromelin, papain, and trypsine soften and aid in the hydration of the skin?
   a. by dissolving collagen   c. by dissolving keratin
   b. by hardening collagen   d. by hardening keratin _____

13. What is particularly suited to presurgical treatment because of its gentle hydrating and exfoliating benefits?
   a. microdermabrasion   c. microcurrent
   b. enzyme peel   d. ultrasonic _____

14. What purpose do AHAs, allantoin, BHAs, chamomile, and enzymes serve in presurgery home care kits?
   a. exfoliation   c. moisturization
   b. cleansing   d. sun protection _____

15. What treatment has muscle strengthening aspects that can be intermixed with other treatments to help condition and tone the skin before surgical or laser intervention?
    a. microcurrent facial toning
    b. lymph drainage
    c. microdermabrasion
    d. ultrasonic treatment
    _____

16. How often will you need to see the client for microcurrent facial toning in the period immediately after surgery?
    a. on a daily basis
    b. at least twice weekly
    c. on a weekly basis
    d. at least twice monthly
    _____

17. What is **NOT** true of lymph drainage?
    a. it stimulates fluid movement
    b. it reduces inflammation
    c. it increases muscle tension
    d. it increases relaxation
    _____

18. How far apart should lymph drainage treatments be spaced?
    a. two weeks to 20 days
    b. one to two weeks
    c. four days to one week
    d. two to three days
    _____

19. What offers a deep relaxation not offered by other types of massage?
    a. manual lymph drainage
    b. microdermabrasion
    c. petrissage
    d. tapotement
    _____

20. When should you provide the **LAST** presurgical treatment?
    a. three hours before the procedure
    b. three days before the procedure
    c. six hours before the procedure
    d. six days before the procedure
    _____

21. What is found in the doctor-provided kits that clients use when receiving laser treatments, but **NOT** found in the kits for clients receiving other medical procedures?
    a. Dysport
    b. arnica montana
    c. hydroquinone
    d. Botox Cosmetic
    _____

22. What is **NOT** true about products used for the treatment of patients with cancer?
    a. they should be gentle
    b. they should be intended for sensitive skin
    c. they should be fragrance-free
    d. they should be intended for couperose skin
    _____

23. What purpose does hydroquinone serve in a prelaser home care kit?
    a. moisturization   c. skin-lightening
    b. sun protection   d. exfoliation   _____

24. What should you get before performing any postprocedure treatments?
    a. permission from the state health department
    b. permission from the state medical board
    c. salon manager's approval
    d. physician's approval   _____

25. What medication is **NOT** commonly prescribed for patients after procedures?
    a. Zyrtec   c. Famvir
    b. Zithromax Z Pak   d. Valtrex   _____

26. What part of the skin may be impaired after laser resurfacing procedures, inhibiting normal response to either heat or cold?
    a. collagen   c. hair follicles
    b. nerve endings   d. elastin   _____

27. How soon after laser resurfacing treatment does reepithelization, the regrowth of skin, generally occur?
    a. immediately
    b. between three and 14 hours
    c. between three and 14 days
    d. between 14 days and one month   _____

28. What can happen easily during reepithelization if the esthetician is not careful?
    a. hyperpigmentation   c. loss of vellus hairs
    b. loss of terminal hairs   d. skin trauma   _____

29. How often should the postprocedure patient apply solution soaks to the skin after removal of the dressing?
    a. every two to three hours c. twice a day
    b. every six to eight hours d. once a day   _____

30. What is a priority when treating postprocedure skin after laser treatments?
    a. keeping the skin warm   c. keeping the skin cool
    b. keeping the skin lubricated d. keeping the skin dry   _____

31. What is **NOT** a warning sign of infection after a procedure?
    a. edema   c. fatigue
    b. oozing   d. eruptions   _____

32. What should be the focus for all treatments during the first three to six months after a laser procedure?
    a. massage and toning
    b. exfoliating and cleansing
    c. extractions and hair removal
    d. hydrating and soothing   _____

33. What term refers to a supportive device worn after surgery of the chin or neck area?
    a. chin/neck bra   c. neck/chin supporter
    b. chin/neck harness   d. neck/chin shield   _____

34. What is a laser procedure that involves vaporization of the epidermis and/or dermis for facial rejuvenation?
    a. laser microdermabrasion   c. laser toning
    b. laser resurfacing   d. laser extraction   _____

35. What is an antiviral medication used to stop or shorten a recurrent outbreak of herpes simplex?
    a. Zithromax Z Pak   c. Valtrex
    b. Aquaphor   d. Famvir   _____

Part 7: Business Skills

CHAPTER 29—FINANCIAL BUSINESS SKILLS

1. What is **NOT** among the new business models that have emerged in the business of skin care during the past two decades?
   - a. massage parlors
   - b. fitness facilities
   - c. medical esthetic practices
   - d. wellness centers
   _____

2. What do you need in order to compete in the modern skin care environment?
   - a. celebrity endorsements
   - b. excellent business and financial management skills
   - c. billionaire investors
   - d. extensive experience in advertising and marketing
   _____

3. What are crucial for obtaining loans to purchase equipment or expand your business?
   - a. investing skills
   - b. advertising skills
   - c. financial skills
   - d. marketing skills
   _____

4. Why does starting a business involve a significant degree of risk?
   - a. new businesses are targeted for arson, theft, and other crimes
   - b. every new business goes through a costly IRS audit in its first year
   - c. the time you invest in your new business will damage your health
   - d. there is no guarantee of a return on your investment
   _____

5. What is **NOT** among the steps you should take prior to opening your own business?
   - a. make promises about profits
   - b. study economic conditions
   - c. analyze the competition
   - d. examine industry trends
   _____

6. What part of a business plan should be written **LAST**?
   - a. marketing plan
   - b. executive summary
   - c. financial plan
   - d. mission statement
   _____

7. What is **NOT** an example of the background information that gives the reader confidence when it is included in an executive summary?
   - a. industry experience
   - b. education
   - c. personal hobbies
   - d. certification
   _____

8. What is a bank representative's main concern when reading a business plan for a salon?
   a. services offered at the salon
   b. types of products sold at the salon
   c. owner's writing skills
   d. owner's ability to repay loans   _____

9. What information does a private investor hope to derive from reading a business plan?
   a. potential return on investment
   b. opportunities for discounted products
   c. opportunities for discounted services
   d. job openings   _____

10. What are advertising, direct marketing, personal selling skills, publicity, public relations, and sales promotions used to develop?
    a. personal friendships   c. employee retention
    b. brand recognition   d. venture capital   _____

11. What is **NOT** one of the four Ps that you should include in your strategic design?
    a. product   c. preparation
    b. price   d. promotion   _____

12. What part of your business plan includes a complete description of your facility and the products and services you will offer, along with realistic goals and objectives?
    a. financial plan   c. mission statement
    b. executive summary   d. strategic plan   _____

13. What is **NOT** found in the operations plan section of a business plan?
    a. schedule for sales promotions
    b. accounting method for the business
    c. designation of managerial responsibility
    d. technology for scheduling appointments   _____

14. What is the single **MOST** important factor in any business plan?
    a. bold mission statement
    b. solid financial strategy
    c. persuasive executive summary
    d. exciting marketing plan   _____

15. What is one of the reasons you should expect to invest personal money in your own business?
    a. to ensure tax deductions that help you hold onto profits
    b. to justify paying yourself a large salary from investors' money
    c. to demonstrate that you are willing to take a risk on yourself
    d. to justify filing for bankruptcy if the business fails _____

16. What can place your business in serious financial jeopardy?
    a. replacing outdated equipment
    b. tying pay increases to profitability
    c. paying bonuses to top workers
    d. falling behind on loan payments _____

17. What is an expectation that venture capitalists generally have in exchange for investing in a business?
    a. some measure of control over the way a business is conducted
    b. the use of their family name as the name of the business
    c. entitlement to free products and services for family and friends
    d. guaranteed payback even if the business fails _____

18. What is a viable path toward additional startup resources for those who qualify?
    a. corporate donations   c. corporate endorsements
    b. government grants   d. government contracts _____

19. How many months of your estimated future pay and/or monthly draw should you include in your application for a business loan?
    a. two   c. 12
    b. six   d. 36 _____

20. What is **NOT** an example of an asset?
    a. facial lounges   c. fixtures
    b. equipment   d. mission statement _____

21. What is typically referred to as the "net worth" of a business?
    a. owner's equity   c. gross profit
    b. liability   d. cost of goods sold _____

22. What is also referred to as a "profit and loss statement"?
    a. financial plan   c. balance sheet
    b. income statement   d. executive summary _____

23. What is the appropriate action for a business with negative cash flow to take?
    a. ask employees to work without pay
    b. speed up purchases of new equipment
    c. borrow money to meet expenses
    d. temporarily stop paying bills _____

24. What do most businesses strive to maintain?
    a. low gross profit
    b. high liabilities
    c. negative cash flow
    d. positive cash flow _____

25. What is a lengthy and arduous task that you may be tempted to forgo, but that you should perform anyway?
    a. conducting a break-even analysis
    b. building salon equipment
    c. formulating pharmaceuticals
    d. conducting door-to-door marketing _____

26. What is the first rule of prevention in any risk management program?
    a. hiring security personnel
    b. strict adherence to guidelines
    c. video monitoring of employees
    d. asking clients to waive liability _____

27. What should you conduct periodically to ensure public safety?
    a. credit checks for vendors
    b. drug tests for employees
    c. safety checks of the entire facility
    d. background checks of clients _____

28. Who is responsible for ensuring that every service provider working in a place of business is licensed by the appropriate state licensing board?
    a. state licensing board representative
    b. service provider
    c. business investors
    d. business owner _____

29. What term refers to the transfer of risk to a third party?
    a. insurance
    b. liability
    c. break-even
    d. venture capital _____

30. What type of insurance is required by law in all states?
    a. rent guarantee
    b. worker's compensation
    c. casualty
    d. kidnap and ransom _____

31. What are some insurance companies now requiring before issuing insurance for certain advanced skin care or hair removal equipment?
    a. photos of equipment placement
    b. samples of marketing materials
    c. proof of adequate training
    d. guarantee of interested clientele ____

32. What should you ask insurance companies for while you are deciding which company to use?
    a. information about competitors
    b. capital for your business
    c. money-back guarantees
    d. client referrals ____

33. What system may **NOT** be in the best interest of salon owners who wish to build a team-based business?
    a. independent contractor   c. salary only
    b. commission only   d. salary plus commission ____

34. What organization is the **BEST** source of information about how tips are taxed?
    a. Small Business Administration (SBA)
    b. Internal Revenue Service (IRS)
    c. American Association for Esthetics (AAE)
    d. Aesthetics International Association (AIA) ____

35. What is **NOT** true about independent contractors, according to the IRS?
    a. they control their own hours
    b. they set their own fees
    c. they cannot accept tips
    d. they pay their own taxes ____

CHAPTER 30—MARKETING

1. What drives business?
   - a. marketing
   - b. training
   - c. scheduling
   - d. licensing _____

2. What term refers to the four Ps (product, price, promotion, and place)?
   - a. marketing bundle
   - b. marketing mix
   - c. advertising bundle
   - d. advertising mix _____

3. What is **NOT** part of the meaning of the word *product*, as it is used in marketing?
   - a. ingredients used for services
   - b. products displayed on retail shelves
   - c. location of your salon
   - d. your menu of services _____

4. Who is involved in the mutually beneficial exchange that forms the basis of marketing?
   - a. employee and proprietor
   - b. business owner and investor
   - c. student and teacher
   - d. buyer and seller _____

5. What is essential to operations and is especially important in building client confidence?
   - a. capable staff
   - b. eye-catching logo
   - c. exciting ad slogan
   - d. celebrity endorsement _____

6. What term refers to the public identification that a business develops through the use of factors including the company's image?
   - a. sales promotion
   - b. brand recognition
   - c. direct marketing
   - d. product analysis _____

7. What should be calculated according to the cost associated with providing a specific service?
   - a. place
   - b. promotion
   - c. price
   - d. product _____

8. What is an example of an indirect cost associated with performing a service?
   - a. labor
   - b. time
   - c. materials
   - d. rent _____

9. What term refers to the way your fees compare with the fees charged by your competitors?
   a. price position
   b. price targeting
   c. fee position
   d. fee targeting _____

10. What is a recommended schedule for implementing each new phase of a carefully planned promotional strategy?
    a. every six to eight days
    b. every six to eight weeks
    c. every six to eight months
    d. every six to eight years _____

11. What tool provides a great way to start looking at the best products and services for your market?
    a. public relations
    b. personal selling
    c. demographics
    d. advertising _____

12. What is a great place to start when you are investigating the demographic resources available to you in your community?
    a. your closest beauty school
    b. your nearby competitors
    c. your state licensing board
    d. your local chamber of commerce _____

13. What information is **NOT** commonly collected during independent surveys of salon customers?
    a. what foods they eat
    b. what TV shows they watch
    c. what social media they use
    d. what magazines they read _____

14. What is an important part of building a successful sales program that meets clients' needs and satisfies business objectives?
    a. stocking only expensive products
    b. understanding client spending habits
    c. offering only costly services
    d. understanding client exercise habits _____

15. What aspect of a product or service is created by weighing important considerations such as positioning and pricing?
    a. demographic value
    b. demographic promotion
    c. strategic value
    d. strategic promotion _____

16. What is a good exercise for learning how to identify the strategic value of a product?
    a. seeing how the product looks on various different retail shelves
    b. carefully studying the ingredient list on the packaging
    c. watching coupon fliers to see how frequently the product is discounted
    d. asking yourself how you would communicate benefits to a client ____

17. What must salon owners recognize as the most valuable asset in any business?
    a. customers   c. retail products
    b. employees   d. salon equipment ____

18. What is a critical factor in the current marketing environment?
    a. hiring attractive receptionists
    b. maintaining quality control
    c. advertising exclusively on radio
    d. rushing clients through services ____

19. Who in the salon must be invested in developing positive customer relationships?
    a. only the estheticians   c. everyone in the salon
    b. only the receptionist   d. only the management ____

20. What is generally considered the least expensive type of advertising?
    a. television ads   c. Internet ads
    b. radio ads   d. classified ads ____

21. What form of advertising can be helpful in building name recognition and defining a salon's image, even though the prices for ads can be high?
    a. magazine   c. e-mail
    b. classified   d. direct mail ____

22. What form of advertising requires continuity in order to be effective?
    a. classified   c. magazine
    b. television   d. e-mail ____

23. What is the key to successful and cost-effective direct-mail efforts?
    a. hiring a celebrity spokesperson
    b. sending out new mailers every day
    c. maintaining an up-to-date database
    d. mailing to every person in your city ____

24. What term refers to an internal marketing method meant to retain valued clients?
    a. direct marketing
    b. sales promotions
    c. personal selling
    d. rewards programs
    ____

25. What is critical to evaluating the success of any advertising and/or marketing effort?
    a. tracking results
    b. making sure the media outlet you used is satisfied
    c. confirming that your ads appear
    d. making sure your employees liked the ad campaign
    ____

26. What is the **MOST** involved method of promotion available to small-business owners?
    a. rewards programs
    b. public relations
    c. sales promotions
    d. direct marketing
    ____

27. What is **NOT** considered an element of public relations?
    a. advertorials
    b. press releases
    c. incentives
    d. media kits
    ____

28. Why do public-relations professionals encourage business owners to perform good work and plan events?
    a. to increase fees paid to PR firms
    b. to give business owners tax deductions
    c. to cover up bad business practices
    d. to raise community awareness
    ____

29. What is a caring way to become familiar with local citizens and to let them know a business owner is interested in giving something back to the community?
    a. volunteering services to promote worthy causes
    b. sending direct-mail materials to everyone in the community
    c. hiring a highly skilled worker who happens to be disabled
    d. handing out business cards at local sporting events
    ____

30. What is **NOT** a way to boost a salon's public image and possibly encourage people to patronize the salon?
    a. conducting a skin care class
    b. adding a new service to the menu
    c. helping a local theater group
    d. speaking to a local organization
    ____

31. What is **NOT** an example of direct marketing?
    a. coupons
    c. advertorials
    b. postcards
    d. sales letters ____

32. What are the two important factors of a successful direct marketing campaign?
    a. price and product
    b. medium and message
    c. logo and slogan
    d. offer and target audience ____

33. What is an example of a direct-marketing technique that has been used excessively, prompting many recipients to join registries that protect them from this technique?
    a. telemarketing
    c. radio advertising
    b. TV advertising
    d. classified ads ____

34. What should you do if you send out electronic contacts?
    a. demand an immediate response
    b. make it easy for the client to unsubscribe
    c. send a new message every day
    d. use a deceptive subject line ____

35. Why do skin care professionals have a tremendous advantage over other types of professionals when it comes to personal selling?
    a. skin care professionals can take advantage of client relaxation
    b. skin care professionals can prey upon client insecurity
    c. skin care professionals work closely with clients
    d. skin care professionals do not have this type of advantage ____

Part 1: Orientation

CHAPTER 1—CHANGES IN ESTHETICS

1. a	8. a	15. a	22. c	29. b
2. b	9. b	16. b	23. a	30. a
3. c	10. d	17. c	24. a	31. c
4. d	11. b	18. b	25. a	32. b
5. a	12. b	19. d	26. c	33. b
6. b	13. d	20. a	27. a	34. c
7. d	14. d	21. b	28. b	35. c

Part 2: General Sciences

CHAPTER 2—INFECTION CONTROL

1. c	8. b	15. a	22. a	29. d
2. b	9. c	16. d	23. a	30. a
3. b	10. d	17. b	24. b	31. b
4. c	11. b	18. a	25. c	32. d
5. d	12. a	19. d	26. d	33. c
6. c	13. a	20. c	27. b	34. d
7. a	14. d	21. b	28. c	35. b

CHAPTER 3—ADVANCED HISTOLOGY OF THE CELL AND THE SKIN

1. a	8. a	15. a	22. a	29. d
2. b	9. d	16. d	23. b	30. d
3. c	10. a	17. a	24. a	31. a
4. d	11. b	18. b	25. d	32. d
5. a	12. b	19. c	26. c	33. d
6. b	13. d	20. a	27. b	34. a
7. b	14. c	21. b	28. c	35. c

CHAPTER 4—HORMONES

1. a	8. d	15. a	22. d	29. c
2. b	9. a	16. b	23. a	30. d
3. c	10. b	17. c	24. b	31. a
4. d	11. a	18. d	25. c	32. b
5. a	12. d	19. a	26. d	33. c
6. a	13. b	20. b	27. a	34. d
7. b	14. b	21. c	28. b	35. a

CHAPTER 5—ANATOMY AND PHYSIOLOGY: MUSCLES AND NERVES

1. a	8. d	15. b	22. a	29. d
2. b	9. a	16. c	23. b	30. a
3. c	10. b	17. d	24. c	31. b
4. a	11. c	18. a	25. d	32. c
5. d	12. d	19. b	26. a	33. d
6. b	13. a	20. c	27. b	34. a
7. c	14. a	21. d	28. c	35. c

CHAPTER 6—ANATOMY AND PHYSIOLOGY: THE CARDIOVASCULAR AND LYMPHATIC SYSTEMS

1. a	8. d	15. c	22. c	29. a
2. b	9. a	16. d	23. d	30. b
3. c	10. b	17. b	24. a	31. c
4. d	11. c	18. c	25. b	32. d
5. a	12. d	19. d	26. a	33. a
6. b	13. a	20. a	27. c	34. b
7. c	14. b	21. b	28. d	35. c

CHAPTER 7—CHEMISTRY AND BIOCHEMISTRY

1. a	8. d	15. c	22. b	29. a
2. b	9. a	16. d	23. c	30. b
3. c	10. b	17. a	24. d	31. b
4. d	11. c	18. b	25. a	32. c
5. a	12. d	19. c	26. b	33. d
6. b	13. a	20. d	27. c	34. a
7. c	14. b	21. a	28. d	35. b

CHAPTER 8—LASER, LIGHT ENERGY, AND RADIOFREQUENCY THERAPY

1. a	8. d	15. c	22. b	29. a
2. b	9. a	16. d	23. c	30. b
3. c	10. b	17. a	24. d	31. c
4. d	11. c	18. b	25. a	32. d
5. a	12. d	19. c	26. b	33. a
6. b	13. a	20. d	27. c	34. b
7. c	14. b	21. a	28. d	35. c

Part 3: Skin Sciences

CHAPTER 9—WELLNESS MANAGEMENT

1. a	8. a	15. a	22. c	29. d
2. b	9. b	16. b	23. d	30. d
3. c	10. b	17. c	24. d	31. a
4. a	11. b	18. c	25. c	32. b
5. a	12. c	19. b	26. a	33. c
6. d	13. d	20. a	27. b	34. d
7. d	14. b	21. b	28. c	35. a

CHAPTER 10—ADVANCED SKIN DISORDERS: SKIN IN DISTRESS

1. a	8. c	15. c	22. d	29. b
2. d	9. d	16. a	23. b	30. c
3. c	10. c	17. d	24. a	31. d
4. d	11. a	18. a	25. b	32. a
5. a	12. b	19. b	26. b	33. c
6. d	13. c	20. c	27. b	34. d
7. b	14. b	21. c	28. a	35. a

CHAPTER 11—SKIN TYPING AND AGING ANALYSIS

1. d	8. c	15. d	22. b	29. a
2. a	9. b	16. a	23. c	30. b
3. a	10. d	17. d	24. d	31. d
4. b	11. a	18. b	25. a	32. c
5. c	12. c	19. d	26. b	33. a
6. a	13. b	20. c	27. d	34. b
7. b	14. c	21. a	28. c	35. b

CHAPTER 12—SKIN CARE PRODUCTS: CHEMISTRY, INGREDIENTS, AND SELECTION

1. a	8. c	15. b	22. a	29. d
2. b	9. d	16. c	23. b	30. a
3. c	10. c	17. d	24. c	31. b
4. d	11. a	18. a	25. d	32. c
5. a	12. b	19. b	26. a	33. d
6. b	13. d	20. c	27. b	34. a
7. c	14. a	21. d	28. c	35. b

CHAPTER 13—BOTANICALS AND AROMATHERAPY

1. a	8. c	15. c	22. d	29. a
2. b	9. b	16. d	23. b	30. d
3. c	10. c	17. a	24. a	31. d
4. b	11. d	18. a	25. b	32. a
5. d	12. a	19. b	26. c	33. a
6. a	13. d	20. b	27. c	34. b
7. c	14. b	21. c	28. d	35. c

CHAPTER 14—INGREDIENTS AND PRODUCTS FOR SKIN ISSUES

1. a	8. d	15. c	22. b	29. a
2. b	9. a	16. d	23. c	30. b
3. c	10. b	17. a	24. d	31. c
4. d	11. c	18. b	25. c	32. d
5. a	12. d	19. c	26. a	33. a
6. b	13. a	20. d	27. b	34. b
7. c	14. b	21. a	28. d	35. c

CHAPTER 15—PHARMACOLOGY FOR ESTHETICIANS

1. a	8. d	15. c	22. d	29. d
2. b	9. a	16. a	23. a	30. a
3. c	10. b	17. b	24. b	31. b
4. d	11. c	18. c	25. c	32. c
5. a	12. d	19. d	26. a	33. d
6. b	13. a	20. a	27. b	34. a
7. c	14. b	21. c	28. c	35. b

Part 4: Advanced Esthetics

CHAPTER 16—ADVANCED FACIAL TECHNIQUES

1. b	8. b	15. c	22. b	29. a
2. a	9. c	16. d	23. c	30. b
3. b	10. d	17. a	24. d	31. c
4. c	11. d	18. b	25. a	32. d
5. d	12. a	19. c	26. b	33. a
6. c	13. a	20. d	27. c	34. b
7. a	14. b	21. a	28. d	35. c

CHAPTER 17—ADVANCED SKIN CARE MASSAGE

1. a	8. d	15. c	22. b	29. a
2. b	9. a	16. d	23. c	30. b
3. c	10. b	17. a	24. d	31. d
4. a	11. c	18. b	25. a	32. c
5. a	12. d	19. c	26. b	33. a
6. b	13. a	20. d	27. c	34. b
7. c	14. b	21. a	28. d	35. c

CHAPTER 18—ADVANCED FACIAL DEVICES

1. a	8. d	15. c	22. b	29. a
2. b	9. a	16. d	23. c	30. b
3. c	10. b	17. a	24. d	31. c
4. d	11. c	18. b	25. a	32. d
5. a	12. d	19. c	26. b	33. a
6. b	13. a	20. d	27. c	34. b
7. c	14. b	21. a	28. d	35. c

CHAPTER 19—ADVANCED HAIR REMOVAL

1. a	8. d	15. c	22. b	29. a
2. b	9. a	16. d	23. d	30. b
3. c	10. b	17. a	24. c	31. c
4. d	11. c	18. b	25. a	32. d
5. a	12. d	19. d	26. b	33. a
6. b	13. a	20. c	27. c	34. b
7. c	14. b	21. a	28. d	35. c

CHAPTER 20—ADVANCED MAKEUP

1. a	8. d	15. c	22. b	29. a
2. c	9. a	16. d	23. c	30. b
3. b	10. b	17. a	24. d	31. c
4. c	11. c	18. b	25. a	32. d
5. d	12. d	19. c	26. b	33. a
6. a	13. a	20. d	27. c	34. b
7. b	14. b	21. a	28. d	35. c

Part 5: Spa and Alternative Therapies

CHAPTER 21—SPA TREATMENTS

1. a	8. d	15. a	22. c	29. b
2. b	9. c	16. b	23. d	30. c
3. c	10. d	17. b	24. a	31. d
4. d	11. a	18. a	25. c	32. a
5. a	12. b	19. d	26. d	33. b
6. b	13. c	20. a	27. a	34. c
7. c	14. d	21. b	28. b	35. c

CHAPTER 22—COMPLEMENTARY WELLNESS THERAPIES

1. a	8. d	15. c	22. a	29. d
2. b	9. a	16. d	23. b	30. b
3. c	10. b	17. a	24. d	31. c
4. d	11. c	18. b	25. a	32. d
5. a	12. d	19. c	26. b	33. a
6. b	13. a	20. d	27. c	34. b
7. c	14. b	21. c	28. b	35. c

CHAPTER 23—AYURVEDA THEORY AND TREATMENTS

1. a	8. d	15. a	22. b	29. c
2. b	9. a	16. b	23. d	30. d
3. c	10. c	17. c	24. d	31. a
4. c	11. d	18. d	25. a	32. b
5. b	12. d	19. a	26. c	33. a
6. c	13. c	20. a	27. b	34. b
7. d	14. a	21. b	28. b	35. c

Part 6: Medical Sciences

CHAPTER 24—WORKING IN A MEDICAL SETTING

1. a	8. d	15. c	22. b	29. a
2. b	9. a	16. c	23. c	30. b
3. c	10. b	17. d	24. d	31. c
4. d	11. c	18. a	25. a	32. d
5. a	12. d	19. b	26. b	33. a
6. b	13. a	20. c	27. c	34. b
7. c	14. b	21. d	28. d	35. c

CHAPTER 25—MEDICAL TERMINOLOGY

1. a	8. d	15. c	22. b	29. c
2. b	9. a	16. c	23. b	30. c
3. c	10. b	17. d	24. c	31. b
4. a	11. a	18. a	25. c	32. d
5. a	12. a	19. d	26. d	33. b
6. d	13. b	20. a	27. b	34. d
7. c	14. a	21. b	28. d	35. c

CHAPTER 26—MEDICAL INTERVENTION

1. a	8. c	15. d	22. c	29. c
2. b	9. d	16. a	23. d	30. b
3. c	10. a	17. a	24. a	31. c
4. d	11. b	18. c	25. c	32. d
5. a	12. d	19. d	26. d	33. a
6. b	13. b	20. a	27. a	34. b
7. b	14. c	21. b	28. b	35. c

CHAPTER 27—PLASTIC SURGERY PROCEDURES

1. a	8. d	15. c	22. b	29. a
2. b	9. a	16. d	23. c	30. b
3. c	10. b	17. a	24. d	31. c
4. d	11. c	18. b	25. a	32. d
5. a	12. d	19. c	26. c	33. a
6. b	13. b	20. d	27. b	34. b
7. c	14. b	21. a	28. d	35. c

CHAPTER 28—THE ESTHETICIAN'S ROLE IN PRE- AND POST-MEDICAL TREATMENTS

1. a	8. c	15. a	22. d	29. a
2. b	9. d	16. b	23. c	30. b
3. c	10. a	17. c	24. d	31. c
4. d	11. b	18. d	25. a	32. d
5. a	12. c	19. a	26. b	33. a
6. a	13. d	20. b	27. c	34. b
7. b	14. b	21. c	28. d	35. c

Part 7: Business Skills

CHAPTER 29—FINANCIAL BUSINESS SKILLS

1. a	8. d	15. c	22. b	29. a
2. b	9. a	16. d	23. c	30. b
3. c	10. b	17. a	24. d	31. c
4. d	11. c	18. b	25. a	32. d
5. a	12. d	19. c	26. b	33. a
6. b	13. a	20. d	27. c	34. b
7. c	14. b	21. a	28. d	35. c

CHAPTER 30—MARKETING

1. a	8. d	15. c	22. b	29. a
2. b	9. a	16. d	23. c	30. b
3. c	10. b	17. a	24. d	31. c
4. d	11. c	18. b	25. a	32. d
5. a	12. d	19. c	26. b	33. a
6. b	13. a	20. d	27. c	34. b
7. c	14. b	21. a	28. d	35. c